Official Journal of the Collegium Internationale Allergologicum

International Archives of Allergy and Immunology

Founded 1950 by D. Harley, P. Kallós, W. Löffler and F.W. Wittich
Continued by E.A. Brown (1952–1954), W. Kaufman (1955–1967),
F. Hahn (1961–1972), H.C. Goodman (1963–1975),
R.R.A. Coombs (1955–1984), Z. Trnka (1972–1987), P. Kallós (1950–1988),
G.B. West (1959–1991), J. Bienenstock (1990–1991), L.Å. Hanson (1981–1991),
K. Kano (1982–1991), F. Milgrom (1965–1991), K. Rother (1982–1991),
G. Wick (1991–1997), B. Grubeck-Loebenstein (1991–1997)

KARGER

Printed in Switzerland
on acid-free paper by
Reinhardt Druck, Basel

Appears monthly:
3 volumes per year
(12 issues)

Guidelines for Authors

International Archives of
Allergy and
Immunology

'International Archives of Allergy and Immunology' appears monthly and provides a forum for publication of work from all aspects of modern allergology and immunology. Papers considered of special interest will be treated as 'hot topics' and every attempt will be made to publish these especially fast. Starting in 1998, a new Editor-in-Chief, Managing Editor and a team of internationally established Associate Editors competently covering all fields of allergology and immunology will be responsible for the scientific quality of this international core journal. *International Archives* will publish original work in the fields of allergy, immunopathology and transplantation, cellular immunology, immunogenetics, immunopharmacology and immunoendocrinology, mucosal immunity, immunology of infectious diseases and immunology of connective tissue diseases. In addition, reviews, minireviews, commentaries and opinions on controversial subjects will be published regularly. A new system of manuscript submission, reviewing and processing will guarantee competent and fair reviewing as well as fast and high quality publication.

Submission

Only papers written in English are considered. Manuscripts should be submitted in triplicate (with three sets of illustrations of which one is an original), typewritten double-spaced on one side of the paper, with a wide margin. The papers should be sent to:

Prof. Dr. D. Kraft
Editor-in-Chief
S. Karger AG
Editorial Office International Archives of
Allergy and Immunology
P.O. Box
CH–4009 Basel (Switzerland)
Telephone +41 61 306 1360
Fax +41 61 306 1434
E-mail e.lieberherr@karger.ch

Mailing address for courier deliveries only:

Allschwilerstr. 10
CH–4055 Basel (Switzerland)

Original research papers: Submitted manuscripts should be fully documented reports of original research. They must describe significant and original observations to be critically evaluated and, if necessary, repeated.

Short communications: These manuscripts should not contain more than **2 printed pages (i.e. 5 manuscript pages)**, including an abstract, essential references and not more than 3 tables or figures. Such communications should represent complete, original studies and should be arranged in the same way as full length manuscripts.

Case reports of general immunological interest can be submitted.

Review articles, minireviews and commentaries: Authors, who wish to contribute a manuscript to one of these categories should contact the Editor-in-Chief. Minireviews should be focused, brief reports on topics of current interest. Commentaries should offer a more personalized perspective on a topic that will be of interest to the general readership. All contributions to these categories will be subject to Editorial review.

Letters to the Editor concerning work published in the journal may be submitted. They should not exceed 2 manuscript pages including one table or figure.

Conditions

All manuscripts are subject to editorial review. Manuscripts are received with the explicit understanding that they are not under simultaneous consideration by any other publication. A cover letter with the name, address, and telephone and telefax numbers of the corresponding author must accompany each manuscript. This letter must include a statement that affirms that all authors concur with the submission. Submission of an article for publication implies the transfer of the copyright from the author to the publisher upon acceptance. Accepted papers become the permanent property of 'International Archives of Allergy and Immunology' and may not be reproduced by any means, in whole or in part, without the written consent of the publisher. It is the author's responsibility to obtain permission to reproduce illustrations, tables, etc. from other publications. One of the criteria considered in reviewing manuscripts is the proper treatment of animals. In particular, the use of painful or otherwise noxious stimuli must be carefully and thoroughly justified. Papers that do not meet these criteria will not be accepted for publication.

Arrangement

Title page: The first page of each paper should indicate the title (main title underlined), the authors' names, and the institution where the work was conducted. A short title for use as running head is also required.

Key words: A list of 3–10 key words should be included for indexing purposes.

Abstract: **Provide on a separate page an abstract of not more than 250 words. This abstract should consist of four paragraphs, labeled Background, Methods, Results, and Conclusions. They should briefly describe, respectively, the problem being addressed in the study, how the study was performed, the salient results, and what the authors conclude from the results.**
The text should be arranged in the following sections: Introduction, Material and Methods, Results, Discussion, Acknowledgement, References.

Small type: Paragraphs which can or must be set in smaller type (case histories, test methods, etc.) should be indicated with a 'p' (petit) in the margin on the left-hand side.

Footnotes: Avoid footnotes. When essential, they are numbered consecutively and typed at the foot of the appropriate page.

Tables and illustrations: Tables and illustrations (both numbered in Arabic numerals) should be prepared on separate sheets. Tables require a heading and figures a legend, also prepared on a separate sheet. For the reproduction of illustrations, only good drawings and original photographs can be accepted; negatives or photocopies cannot be used. Due to technical reasons, figures with a screen background should not be submitted. When possible, group several illustrations on one block for reproduction (max. size 181 × 223 mm) or provide crop marks. On the back of each illustration, indicate its number, the author's name, and 'top' with a soft pencil.

Color illustrations: Up to 6 color illustrations per page can be integrated with the text at the reduced price of CHF 660.–/USD 545.00 per page. Color illustrations are reproduced at the author's expense.

Abbreviations: Avoid overuse of abbreviations. Introduce an abbreviation only when the same term occurs three or more times.

References: In the text identify references by Arabic numerals [in square brackets]. Material submitted for publication but not yet accepted should be noted as 'unpublished data' and not be included in the reference list. The list of references should include only those publications which are cited in the text. Do not alphabetize; number references in the order in which they are first mentioned in the text. The surnames of the authors followed by initials should be given. There should be no punctuation other than a comma to separate the authors. Cite all authors, 'et al' is not sufficient. Abbreviate journal names according to the Index Medicus system. (Also see International Committee of Medical Journal Editors: Uniform requirements for manuscripts submitted to biomedical journals. N Engl J Med 1997;336:309–315.)

Examples
(a) Papers published in periodicals: Sun J, Koto H, Chung KF: Interaction of ozone and allergen challenges on bronchial responsiveness and inflammation in sensitised guinea pigs. Int Arch Allergy Immunol 1997;112:191–195.
(b) Monographs: Matthews DE, Farewell VT: Using and Understanding Medical Statistics, ed 3, revised. Basel, Karger, 1996.
(c) Edited books: Parren PWHI, Burton DR: Antibodies against HIV-1 from phage display libraries: Mapping of an immune response and progress towards antiviral immunotherapy; in Capra JD (ed): Antibody Engineering. Chem Immunol. Basel, Karger, 1997, vol 65, pp 18–56.

Full address: The exact postal address complete with postal code must be given at the bottom of the title page. Please also supply phone and fax numbers, as well as your e-mail address.

Page charges

There is no page charge for papers of 5 or fewer printed pages (including tables, illustrations and references). Each additional complete or partial page is charged to the author at CHF 275.–/USD 196.–. The allotted size of a paper is equal to approx. 14 manuscript pages (including tables, illustrations and references).

Galley proofs

Unless indicated otherwise, galley proofs are sent to the first-named author and should be returned with the least possible delay. Alterations made in galley proofs, other than the correction of printer's errors, are charged to the author. No page proofs are supplied.

Reprints

Order forms and a price list are sent with the galley proofs. Orders submitted after the issue is printed are subject to considerably higher prices.

KARGER

Fax+41 61 306 12 34
E-Mail karger@karger.ch
www.karger.com

The Guidelines for Authors are available at:
www.karger.com/journals/iaa/iaa_gl.htm

General Information

International Archives of
Allergy and
Immunology

Publication data: 'International Archives of Allergy and Immunology' is published 12 times a year. Volumes 118–120 with 4 issues each appear in 1999.

Subscription rates: Subscriptions run for a full calendar year. Prices are given per volume.
Personal subscription:
Subscription + postage and handling
CHF 397.– + CHF 15.70 Europe
CHF 397.– + CHF 23.70 Overseas
USD 306.00 + USD 15.70
(Must be in the name of, billed to, and paid by an individual. Order must be marked 'personal subscription'.)
Institutional subscription:
Subscription + postage and handling
CHF 794.– + CHF 19.60 Europe
CHF 794.– + CHF 29.60 Overseas
USD 612.00 + USD 19.60
Airmail postage: CHF 24.–, USD 20.00.
(Extra per volume.)
Discount subscription prices:
Subscription + postage and handling
CHF 208.– + CHF 47.10 Europe
CHF 208.– + CHF 71.10 Overseas
USD 159.00 + USD 47.10
Members of following societies: AAAAI, AAI, BSACI, BSI, CSI, CIA, DGAI, DGI, EAACI, EFIS, ÖGAI, SFI, SGAI

Microforms: Please direct all enquiries and orders to: University Microfilms Inc.
300 North Zeeb Road, P.O. Box 1346
Ann Arbor, MI 48106-1346 (USA)

Subscription orders: Orders can be placed at agencies, bookstores, directly with the Publisher
S. Karger AG, P.O. Box,
CH–4009 Basel (Switzerland)
or with any of the following distributors:
Deutschland: S. Karger GmbH, Postfach
D–79095 Freiburg
France: Librairie Luginbühl
36, bd de Latour-Maubourg, F–75007 Paris
Great Britain, Ireland: S. Karger Publishers
58 Grove Hill Road
Tunbridge Wells, Kent TN1 1SP
USA: S. Karger Publishers, Inc.
26 West Avon Road, P.O. Box 529
Farmington, CT 06085
India, Bangladesh, Sri Lanka:
S. Karger India Subscription Agency
B–5/132 Safdarjung Enclave
New Delhi-110029
Japan: Katakura Libri, Inc.
2F, Marushima Bldg, 4-6-17, Yushima,
Bunkyo-ku, Tokyo 113-0034

Change of address: Both old and new address should be sent to the subscription source.

Single issues and back volumes: Information can be obtained through the Publisher.

Advertising: Correspondence and rate requests should be addressed to the Publisher.

Bibliographic indices: This journal is regularly listed in bibliographic services, including *Current Contents®*.

Book Reviews: Books are accepted for review by special agreement.

Copying: This journal has been registered with the Copyright Clearance Center (CCC), as indicated by the code appearing on the first page of each article.
For readers in the US, this code signals consent for copying of articles for personal or internal use, or for the personal or internal use of specific clients, provided that the stated fee is paid per copy directly to
Copyright Clearance Center Inc.
222 Rosewood Drive
Danvers, MA 01923 (USA)
A copy of the first page of the article must accompany payment. Consent does not extend to copying for general distribution, for promotion, for creating new works, or for resale. In these cases, specific written permission must be obtained from the copyright owner,
S. Karger AG,
P.O. Box, CH–4009 Basel (Switzerland).

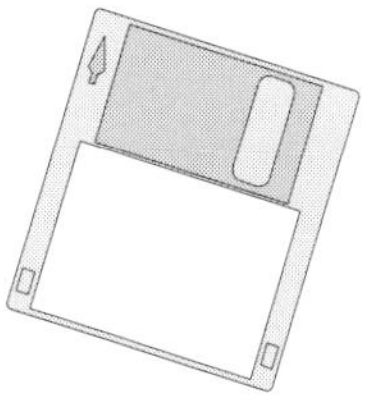

Disk Submission

A **comprehensive version** of these guidelines for the **submission of manuscripts and illustrations on disk** can be accessed online under **www.karger.com/journals/disksub.htm** or requested as a leaflet from the editorial department.

Please follow the general rules on style and arrangement in the **"Guidelines for Authors"** of the journal. Submit a **double-spaced printout** of your manuscript matching the file on disk exactly.

Technical Information

Store only data pertinent to this manuscript. Include your fonts (screen and printer fonts for Macintosh). For a **text only** manuscript, use a 3.5 inch disk. For **text and illustrations,** use 3.5 or 5.25 Magneto Optical Disc; CD-ROM (DOS or hybrid); iomage Zip/DOS (100 MB), or 44 MB, 88 MB or 200 MB SyQuest. Compress extensive data using ZIP format.

Data Description

Label your disk with the **title of the journal or book** for which it is submitted; a **short version** of the paper's title; your **name,** postal and e-mail address, fax and phone number; **hard and software** used, including the version; and the **complete list of the file names.** File names consist of eight characters before the dot identifying the file and three characters after the dot identifying the application.

Text and Format

The **preferred word-processing package is MS-Word.** Other commonly used PC text programs and ASCII formats are accepted.
Update your data when you revise subsequent to the reviewer's or editor's decision and mark revisions clearly. Manuscripts accepted for publication are subject to **copy editing:** changes and/or questions will be marked in the manuscript, which will be returned to you with your disk and the galley proofs for checking.
Enter your text continuously flush left. Do not use any layout functions. Do not split words at the end of a line. **Do not use indentations.** Use a blank line before and a hard return at the end of paragraphs. **Arrange headings flush left.** Insert only **one space after punctuation marks.** Insert Greek letters, mathematical symbols etc. with your word-processing program. Use **boldface and italics** as well as sub- and superscript where appropriate.
Tables are part of the text and should be placed at the end of the text file. Separate the individual parts of a table by lines. Use the tabulator instead of spaces. Format operation data on one line in the same column. **Legends to illustrations are part of the text** and should also be listed at the end of the text file.

Illustrations

Store illustrations as separate files: do not embed them in your text. Export **line drawings/vector graphics** as TIF, EPS or WMF format. Use Photoshop for processing and retouching **scanned halftone images.** Save the original scan and the processed version. Export **black and white or color images** as TIF or EPS format in their anticipated size in print.
For detailed information on how to submit illustration data on disk please consult the leaflet or **www.karger.com/journals/disksub.htm.**

KARGER

Fax +41 61 306 12 34
E-Mail karger@karger.ch
www.karger.com

The Journal Home Page is available at:
www.karger.com/journals/iaa

KI 98 DISK

State-of-the-art reviews by leading experts

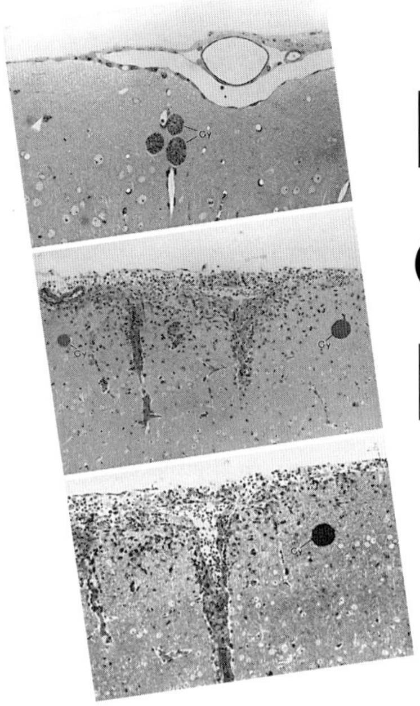

Immunology of Intracellular Parasitism

Editors: Foo Yew Liew, Frank E.G. Cox

Intracellular prokaryotic and eukaryotic organisms cause some of the most intractable problems in the fields of human and animal infectious diseases. Such infections are characteristically long and chronic and accompanied by deleterious immunopathological changes. The nine chapters in this volume, all written by internationally acknowledged experts in their fields, explore the immunological features common to representative intracellular organisms and also the special features whereby particular species evade immune attack and how they are destroyed with special reference to experimental and human listeriosis, tuberculosis, leishmaniasis, toxoplasmosis, African and American trypanosomiasis, malaria, cryptosporidiosis and the cattle disease theileriosis. The emphasis is on the roles of lymphocytes, macrophages, NK cells, cytokines and the contrasting roles of Th1/Th2 cells in protective and counter-protective immune responses. The importance of understanding these phenomena for the development of vaccines, for strategies for ameliorating immunopathological responses and for explaining why some infections are important concomitants in AIDS while others are not is stressed.

This volume brings together and establishes links between diverse studies concerning the immunological aspects of the host-parasite relationship otherwise scattered throughout the literature. Authoritative and up-to-date, it will be of particular interest to anyone working or teaching in the fields of immunology, parasitology, microbiology and infectious diseases.

Contents

Chemical Immunology, Vol. 70
Series Editors: Adorini, L. (Milan); Arai, K. (Tokyo); Berek, C. (Berlin); Capra, J.D. (Oklahoma City, Okla.); Schmitt-Verhulst, A.-M. (Marseille); Waksman, B.H. (New York, N.Y.)
ISSN 1015–0145

Fields of Interest: Immunology; Infectious Diseases; Microbiology; Parasitology, Bacteriology, Tropical Medicine

Immunology of Intracellular Parasitism
Editors: Liew, F.Y. (Glasgow); Cox, F.E.G. (London)
XII + 204 p., 17 fig., 6 tab., hard cover, 1998
Institutions: CHF 227.– / DEM 272.– / USD 197.50
Individuals: CHF 113.50 / DEM 136.– / USD 98.75
Prices subject to change
DEM price for Germany, USD price for USA only
ISBN 3–8055–6621–2

KI 98219

KARGER

International Archives of
Allergy and
Immunology

Eosinophils in Allergy and Related Diseases

Proceedings of a Workshop
Tokyo, Japan, June 20, 1998

Guest Editors
Sohei Makino, Tokyo
Takeru Ishikawa, Kumamoto
Takeshi Fukuda, Tochigi

58 figures, 1 in color, and 9 tables, 1999

KARGER

Basel · Freiburg · Paris · London · New York ·
New Delhi · Bangkok · Singapore · Tokyo · Sydney

S. Karger
Medical and Scientific Publishers
Basel · Freiburg · Paris · London
New York · New Delhi · Bangkok
Singapore · Tokyo · Sydney

Drug Dosage
The authors and the publisher have exerted every effort to ensure that drug selection and dosage set forth in this text are in accord with current recommendations and practice at the time of publication. However, in view of ongoing research, changes in government regulations, and the constant flow of information relating to drug therapy and drug reactions, the reader is urged to check the package insert for each drug for any change in indications and dosage and for added warnings and precautions. This is particularly important when the recommended agent is a new and/or infrequently employed drug.

P.O. Box, CH–4009 Basel (Switzerland)
Printed in Switzerland on acid-free paper by
Reinhardt Druck, Basel
ISBN 3–8055–6992–00

KARGER

Fax+ 41 61 306 12 34
E-Mail karger@karger.ch
www.karger.com

Vol. 120, Suppl. 1, 1999

International Archives of Allergy and Immunology

Contents

KARGER

Fax+ 41 61 306 12 34
E-Mail karger@karger.ch
www.karger.com

Access to full text and tables of contents, including tentative ones for forthcoming issues:
www.karger.com/journals/iaa/iaa_bk.htm

International Archives of
Allergy and Immunology

Int Arch Allergy Immunol 1999;120(suppl 1):1

Preface

Sohei Makino, Tokyo *Takeru Ishikawa,* Kumamoto
Takeshi Fukuda, Tochigi

For the past decade, pharmacological management of atopic diseases including bronchial asthma, allergic rhinitis and atopic dermatitis has shown substantial progress. This success is thought to be derived from the advance in understanding the pathophysiology of these diseases and the development of anti-inflammatory agents and improvement of their use, based on newly discovered mechanisms of the disease. Most of these anti-inflammatory agents inhibit infiltration and activation of eosinophils at the sites of the disease including bronchial mucosa, nasal mucosa and the skin.

In asthma, visits to the emergency department and hospitalization due to asthma exacerbation have decreased dramatically. Asthma has been shown to be a chronic inflammatory disease of the airway associated with infiltration of eosinophils, Th2 and mast cells. Among these cells, eosinophils are effector cells for the inflammation of the airway, inducing not only airway hyperresponsiveness but also remodeling of the airway which also induces persistent airway hyperresponsiveness. Eosinophils migrate into the bronchial wall and are activated there by the cytokines released mainly from Th2 and mast cells in the bronchial wall. Recently bronchial epithelial cells produce cytokines which attract and activate eosinophils including eotaxin, GM-CSF, and IL-16. Such mechanisms may explain the eosinophil infiltration in the bronchial walls in nonatopic asthma patients who do not have IgE antibodies to environmental allergens, but show exactly the same symptoms as atopic asthma patients do. Apparently we need more information on the mechanisms of proliferation, activation, migration and tissue damage of eosinophils for the management of atopic diseases.

The initial workshop on Eosinophils in Allergy and Related Diseases took place in Tokyo in 1991. Since then this workshop has reported on up-to-date research on eosinophils and allergy in Japan. The 1998 workshop was held at the Chiwaki Hall in Suido-bashi in Tokyo, with 30 research reports in the fields of clinical and basic science. The main contents concerned the molecular-cellular aspects of formation, activation and biology of eosinophils in relation to clinics of allergy.

The organizing committee has selected 23 papers out of these treaties for inclusion in these proceedings. Conspicuous among these are papers on the mechanisms of eosinophil activation and the interrelationship among eosinophil function, cell surface substance and cytokines. Many of the reports show the change of such interrelationships in allergic disease including asthma, allergic rhinitis and atopic dermatitis.

Topics include eosinophil chemoattractant production from a variety of cells and their activation of eosinophils, modulation of adhesion molecule expression by cytokines and stimulated adhesion molecules, effects of adhesion molecule stimulation and cytokines on eosinophil functions and intracellular signal transduction, alternation of eosinophil function, cytokine mRNA expression and adhesion molecule expression in allergic disease, and animal models of atopic dermatitis and others. These proceedings cover the current issues on eosinophil research in Japan. We hope it will contribute to the research in this field.

Finally, we wish to express our sincere thanks to Novartis Pharma Ltd. for supporting this workshop and the International Medical Publisher (Tokyo) for compiling these proceedings.

KARGER

Fax + 41 61 306 12 34
E-Mail karger@karger.ch
www.karger.com

1018–2438/99/1205–0001$17.50/0

Accessible online at:
http://BioMedNet.com/karger

International Archives of
Allergy and Immunology

Int Arch Allergy Immunol 1999;120(suppl 1):2–6

Human Umbilical Vein Endothelial Cells Support Interleukin-3- and Interleukin-5-Induced Eosinophil Differentiation from Cord Blood CD34+ Cells

Kenichi Ochiai[a] Miho Omura[b] Akinori Mochizuki[a] Motohiro Ito[c] Hisao Tomioka[a]

Departments of [a]Internal Medicine and [c]Obstetrics and Gynecology, Toho University School of Medicine, Sakura Hospital, Sakura, and [b]Department of Biomolecular Science, Faculty of Science, Toho University, Funabashi, Japan

Key Words

Eosinophil differentiation · Human umbilical vein endothelial cells · CD34+ cell · Stem cell factor · Granulocyte/macrophage colony-stimulating factor

Abstract

Background: Human umbilical vein endothelial cells (HUVEC) are an important source of hematopoietic cytokines, and interleukin-3 (IL-3)- and IL-5-induced eosinophil differentiation from CD34+ cells has been observed. To show the supportive effects of endothelial cells on eosinophil differentiation, we examined the effects of cocultured HUVEC on IL-3 and IL-5-induced eosinophil differentiation from human umbilical cord blood CD34+ cells. ***Methods:*** CD34+ cells were obtained from the heparinized umbilical vein blood of 10 volunteers using a CD34-conjugated magnetic bead positive direct selection procedure. With HUVEC in Transwell, CD34+ cells were then cultured for 14–28 days. In neutralizing experiments on HUVEC-derived cytokines, antibodies to both stem cell factor (SCF) and granulocyte/macrophage colony-stimulating factor (GM-CSF) were added to the cell cultures. ***Results:*** Cocultured HUVEC upregulated IL-3 and IL-5-induced eosinophil differentiation from CD34+ cells on day 28 of culture by 75.0%. The eosinophilopoietic effect of HUVEC was significantly only when the cells were present in the culture from day 15 to day 28. Addition of anti-SCF antibody or anti-GM-CSF monoclonal antibody to the culture significantly suppressed HUVEC-combined IL-3- and IL-5-induced eosinophil differentiation on day 28 of culture by 49.2 and 55.0%, respectively. ***Conclusions:*** These results indicate that several cytokines including GM-CSF and SCF from HUVEC promote IL-3- and IL-5-induced eosinophil differentiation from CD34+ cells.

Introduction

The significance of eosinophils as effector cells in allergic inflammations such as bronchial asthma has been recognized [1]. Therefore, determining the regulatory mechanisms of eosinophil function is important in understanding and treating allergic inflammations. But the heterogeneous character of human peripheral eosinophils is often a large obstacle to precise analysis of the cells [2]. An in vitro system capable of producing a large number of pure eosinophils of identical character might be useful for analysis of eosinophil differentiation and function. It has been

KARGER

Fax +41 61 306 12 34
E-Mail karger@karger.ch
www.karger.com

1018–2438/99/1205–0002$17.50/0

Accessible online at:
http://BioMedNet.com/karger

Kenichi Ochiai, MD, DMsci
Department of Internal Medicine, Toho University School of Medicine
Sakura Hospital, 564-1 Shimoshizu, Sakura City, Chiba, 285-0841 (Japan)
Tel. +81 43 462 8811, ext. 2711, Fax +81 43 463 0450
E-Mail kysotiai@alles.or.jp

reported that interleukin-3 (IL-3), IL-5 and granulocyte/macrophage colony-stimulating factor (GM-CSF) are important in eosinophilopoiesis [3, 4] and several studies demonstrated that, in the presence of recombinant human IL-3 (rhIL-3) and rhIL-5, human eosinophils differentiate in vitro from umbilical cord blood-derived progenitor cells [5]; however, the efficacy of eosinophilopoiesis in the system was not sufficient for precise study of eosinophil function.

It has been shown that cytokines produced by accessory cells and the hematopoietic microenvironment [6] are important in hematopoietic progenitor cell proliferation. Stem cell factor (SCF), a multipotent hematopoietic growth factor for early progenitor cells of different lineages [7–9], is produced by cells in this microenvironment, which include fibroblasts and endothelial cells [10]. But, it is generally difficult to use bone marrow cell lines in a human eosinophilopoiesis system. By contrast, endothelial cells from human umbilical vein endothelial cells (HUVEC) release a number of hematopoietic growth factors including SCF and GM-CSF [11].

In this study, in order to show the supportive effects of endothelial cells on eosinophil differentiation, we examined the effect of HUVEC on the differentiation and proliferation of IL-3- and IL-5-induced eosinophils derived from cord blood CD34+ cells.

Materials and Methods

Cytokines and Antibodies

rhIL-3, rhIL-5, and a neutralizing anti-human SCF antibody were obtained from Genzyme (Boston, Mass., USA). A neutralizing anti-human GM-CSF monoclonal antibody (MoAb; mouse, IgG1) was purchased from R&D Systems (Minneapolis, Minn., USA). Control mouse IgG and sheep IgG were obtained from Cappel Labs (Malvern, Pa., USA).

Enrichment of CD34+ Cells

Heparinized cord blood was drawn from 10 donors who were enrolled in this study after informed consent had been obtained. Enrichment of CD34+ cells was by a two-stage procedure: first, centrifugation through Ficoll-Paque (specific gravity = 1.077 g/ml; Pharmacia) gradients to produce mononuclear cell fractions (interface fraction of Ficoll-Paque, and second, using an MoAb against CD34-conjugated magnetic beads in a positive, direct selection procedure using immunomagnetic beads (Dynabeads, DYNAL, Oslo, Norway). In order to dispose of cell-binding immunomagnetic beads from CD34+ cells, detachable beads were used according to the manufacturer's instructions.

Eosinophil Differentiation from CD34+ Cells

CD34+ cells were then suspended at 5 × 10^4 cells/2 ml in RPMI 1640 medium (GIBCO, Grand Island, N.Y., USA) supplemented with 10% fetal calf serum (FCS, GIBCO) and 2 m*M* *L*-glutamine in the presence of rhIL-3 (10 ng/ml) and rhIL-5 (10 ng/ml) in a 12-well flat-bottomed tissue culture plate (Coaster) at 37 °C for 14–28 days. Half of the culture medium was replaced weekly with freshly prepared medium containing the same concentration of rhIL-3 and rhIL-5. At 7, 14, 21 and 28 days after the culture, total cell numbers and viability of the cells were determined by trypan blue dye exclusion, and a differential cell count was conducted by examining 200 cells stained with Wright-Giemsa solution.

Effect of HUVEC on IL-3- and IL-5-Induced Eosinophil Differentiation

To determine the regulatory role of HUVEC in eosinophilopoiesis, we examined the effect of HUVEC on IL-3- and IL-5-induced eosinophil differentiation from CD34+ cells. HUVEC (3041) were obtained from Clonetics (Walkersville, Md., USA). For coculture with stem cells, the precultured HUVEC were harvested by trypsin digestion, seeded into a gelatin-coated Transwell insert (0.33 cm^2 of polycarbonate membrane with 0.4 μm pores; Corning Costar, Cambridge, Mass., USA), and cultured to confluence. Then, the cultured HUVEC in Transwell were inserted into the IL-3- and IL-5-stimulated CD34+ cell culture well from day 0 to day 28.

Further, to determine whether the acceleration of IL-3- and IL-5-induced eosinophil differentiation is exerted by HUVEC in the early or late differentiation stage of the progenitor cells, we also examined the effects of early and late addition of HUVEC to the eosinophil-induced culture. In these experiments, HUVEC in Transwell were only inserted into the IL-3- and IL-5-stimulated progenitor cell culture well from either day 0 to day 14 or day 14 to day 28.

Effect of Anti-SCF and Anti-GM-CSF Antibodies on HUVEC-Accelerated Eosinophil Differentiation

To determine whether SCF and/or GM-CSF, which might be produced from cocultured HUVEC, play a role in regulating eosinophil differentiation, we examined the effect of antibodies which neutralize SCF and GM-CSF on the induced eosinophil differentiation. Anti-human SCF antibody (10 μg/ml), anti-human GM-CSF MoAb (10 μg/ml) or control IgG (10 μg/ml) were added to the culture medium. On the basis of the results of preliminary experiments and previous reports [12, 13], concentration of the neutrizing antibodies was determined. Half of the culture medium was replaced weekly with freshly prepared medium containing rhIL-3, rhIL-5, and the appropriate antibody.

Statistical Analysis

Data are summarized as mean ± SE. The paired Student t test was used for statistical comparison of the data, and a value of $p < 0.05$ was considered significant.

Results

Synergic Effect of Cocultured HUVEC on IL-3- and IL-5-Induced Eosinophil Differentiation from CD34+ Cord Blood Cells

The time course of IL-3- and IL-5-induced eosinophil differentiation from CD34+ cells with or without HUVEC coculture are shown in figure 1. Eosinophils began to

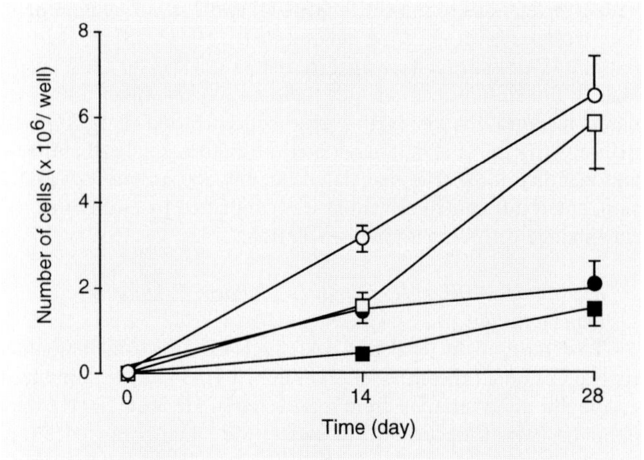

Fig. 1. Time course of IL-3 and IL-5 induced eosinophil differentiation from cord blood CD34+ cells with or without HUVEC. CD34+ cells from human umbilical cord blood (5 × 10^4 cells/2 ml) were cultured in the presence of rhIL-3 (10 ng/ml) and rhIL-5 (10 ng/ml) for 14–28 days. ○ = Total cells with HUVEC; □ = eosinophils with HUVEC; ● = total cells without HUVEC; ■ = eosinophils without HUVEC. Data are means ± SE for 10 experiments.

increase 14 days after culturing CD34+ cells with rhIL-3 and rhIL-5, and cocultured HUVEC significantly enhanced IL-3- and IL-5-induced eosinophil differentiation from the cells on day 28 of culture by 75.0% (n = 10, $p < 0.001$) (fig. 1). The rest of the cultured cells were mainly promyelocytes.

Effect of Cocultured HUVEC on the Late Differentiation Stage of Eosinophil Progenitor Cells

A significant eosinophilopoietic effect was observed when HUVEC was present in the culture from day 15 to day 28 and from day 0 to day 28 (n = 6, $p < 0.05$), whereas HUVEC did not significantly affect eosinophilopoiesis when present in the culture only from day 0 to day 14 (fig. 2).

Effect of Anti-SCF and Anti-GM-CSF MoAb on HUVEC-Enhanced Eosinophil Differentiation

Addition of anti-SCF antibody or anti-GM-CSF MoAb to the culture inhibited HUVEC-enhanced IL-3- and IL-

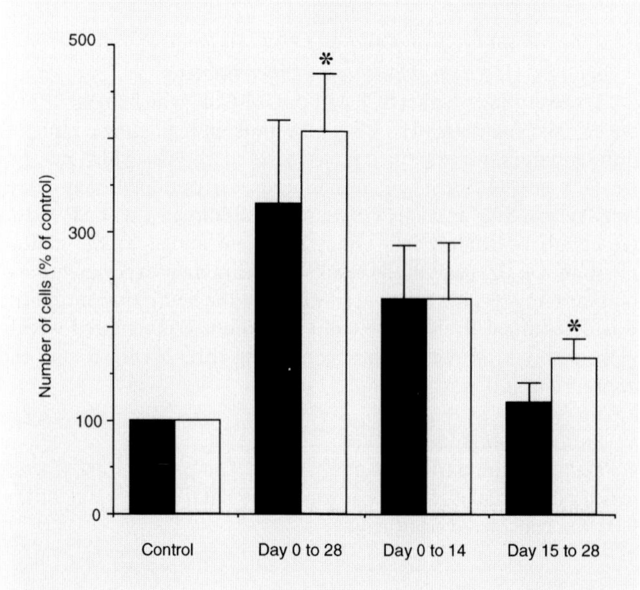

Fig. 2. Effect of late coculture of HUVEC on IL-3 and IL-5 induced eosinophil differentiation from cord blood CD34+ cells. HUVEC in Transwell were cocultured to IL-3- and IL-5-stimulated cord blood CD34+ cells culture from day 0 to day 14 (early coculture) or from day 15 to day 28 (late coculture). ■ = Total cells; □ = eosinophils. The cell number of IL-3 and IL-5 culture without HUVEC is shown as a control. The axis is normalized to the control values. Data are means ± SE for 6 experiments. * $p < 0.05$ vs. mean value of the control response.

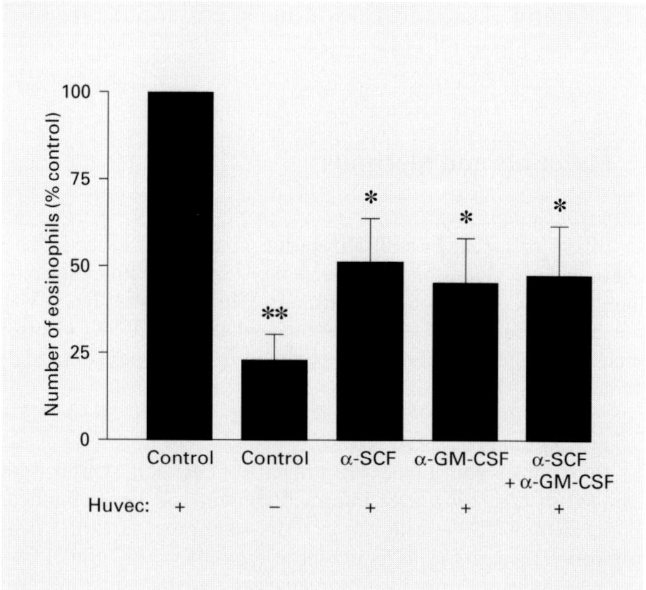

Fig. 3. Effect of anti-SCF and anti-GM-CSF antibodies on IL-3- and IL-5-induced eosinophil differentiation from cord blood CD34+ cells with HUVEC. Anti-SCF antibody (10 μg/ml), anti-GM-CSF MoAb (10 μg/ml) or control IgG (10 μg/ml) were added to IL-3- and IL-5-stimulated cord blood CD34+ cell culture. The number of eosinophils of IL-3 and IL-5 culture with HUVEC and control IgG is shown as a control. The axis is normalized to the control values. Data are means ± SE for 5 experiments. * $p < 0.05$; ** $p < 0.01$ vs. mean value of the control response.

5-induced eosinophil differentiation from CD34+ cells on day 28 of culture by 49.2% ($n = 5$, $p < 0.05$) and 55.0% ($n = 5$, $p < 0.05$), respectively (fig. 3). Combined addition of anti-SCF antibody and anti-GM-CSF MoAb inhibited the eosinophil differentiation significantly (53.2% inhibition, $n = 5$, $p < 0.05$) (fig. 3) but did not completely block the synergetically eosinophilopoietic effect of cocultured HUVEC.

Discussion

In this study, we demonstrated that HUVEC accelerated eosinophil differentiation from CD34+ cells. We found that cocultured HUVEC in Transwell upregulated IL-3- and IL-5-induced eosinophil differentiation from cord blood CD34+ cells (fig. 1). Although the stromal cells may function by direct cell-to-cell contact with hematopoietic cells [14], direct coculture contact between HUVEC and IL-3- and IL-5-induced eosinophils was not examined in order to avoid cell contamination.

We also showed that the supportive effect of HUVEC on eosinophil differentiation was exerted during late stage differentiation. Further, eosinophil differentiation was shown to be significantly inhibited by the addition of neutralizing antibodies for SCF or GM-CSF. HUVEC has been shown to secrete several cytokines, which affect the kinetics of cell cycle-dormant primitive progenitors such as SCF [15] and GM-CSF [16]. SCF is believed to aid in the proliferation of eosinophil precursor cells [17] and to act on late myeloid committed progenitor cells [18]. Therefore, the supportive effect of SCF and GM-SCF from HUVEC appears to be exerted on relatively mature progenitor cells. However, even the combined addition of anti-SCF antibody and anti-GM-CSF MoAb into the culture system failed to completely suppress the enhancement of eosinophil differentiation by HUVEC (fig. 3). HUVEC can also produce IL-6 and IL-8 [19] by several stimulants, but neither IL-6 nor IL-8 is thought to support eosinophilopoiesis [20, 21]. On the other hand, G-CSF is reported to be produced from HUVEC [22] and support the eosinophil differentiation from CD34+ cells [23]. G-CSF might be a third eosinophilopoietic cytokine from cocultured HUVEC.

In conclusion, we have shown that IL-3- and IL-5-induced eosinophil differentiation is upregulated by cytokines secreted from HUVEC.

References

1 Gleich GJ, Flavahan NA, Fujisawa T, Vanhoutte PM: The eosinophil as a mediator of damage to respiratory epithelium: A model for bronchial hyperreactivity. J Allergy Clin Immunol 1988;81:776–781.

2 Hodges MK, Weller PF, Gerard NP, Ackerman SJ, Dtazen JM: Heterogeneity of leukotriene C4 production by eosinophils from asthmatic and from normal subjects. Am Rev Respir Dis 1988;138:799–804.

3 Ogawa M, Katahara T, Leary AG, Sterk AR, Ishizaka K, Ishizaka T: Suspension culture of human mast cells/basophils from umbilical cord blood mononuclear cells. Proc Natl Acad Sci USA 1983;80:4494–4498.

4 Saito H, Hatake K, Dvorak AM, Leifeman KM, Donnenberg AD, Arai N, Ishizaka K, Ishizaka T: Selective differentiation and proliferation of hematopoietic cells induced by recombinant human interleukins. Proc Natl Acad Sci USA 1988;85:2288–2292.

5 Shalit M, Sekhsaria S, Malech HL: Modulation of growth and differentiation of eosinophils from human peripheral blood CD34+ cells by IL5 and other growth factors. Cell Immunol 1995;160:50–57.

6 Carow CE, Hangoc G, Cooper SH, Williams DE: Mast cell growth factor (c-kit ligand) supports the growth of human multipotential progenitor cells with a high replating potential. Blood 1991;78:2216–2221.

7 Zsebo KM, Wypych J, McNiece IK, Lu HS, Smith KA, Karkare SB, Sachdev RK, Yuschenkoff VN, Birkitt NC, Williams LR, et al: Identification of a ligand for the c-kit proto-oncogene. Cell 1990;63:195–201.

8 Williams DE, Eisenman J, Baird A, Rauch C, Van Ness K, March CJ, Park LS, Martin U, Mochizuki DY, Boswell HS, et al: Identification of a ligand for the c-kit proto-oncogene. Cell 1990;63:167–174.

9 Huang E, Nocka K, Beier DR, Chu TY, Buck J, Lahn HW, Wellner D, Leder P, Besmer P: The hematopoietic growth factor KL is encoded by the S1 locus and is the ligand of the c-kit receptor, the gene product of the W locus. Cell 1990; 63:225–233.

10 Aye MT, Hashemi S, Leclair B, Zeibdawi A, Trudel E, Halpenny M, Fuller V, Cheng G: Expression of stem cell factor and c-kit mRNA in cultured endothelial cells, monocytes and cloned human bone marrow stromal cells (CFU-RF). Exp Hematol 1992;20:523–527.

11 Koenig A, Yakisan E, Reuter M, Huang M, Sykora K-W, Corbacioglu S, Welte K: Differential regulation of stem cell factor mRNA expression in human endothelial cells by bacterial pathogens: An in vitro model of inflammation. Blood 1994;83:2836–2843.

12 Zupo S, Perussia B, Baldi L, Coorcione A, Dono M, Ferrarini M, Pistoria V: Production of granulocyte-macrophage colony-stimulating factor but not IL-3 by normal and neoplastic human B lymphocytes. J Immunol 1992;148: 1423–1430.

13 Yamaguchi H, Ishii E, Saito S, Tashiro K, Fujita I, Yoshidomi S, Ohtubo M, Akazawa K, Miyazaki S: Umbilical vein endothelial cells are an important source of c-kit and stem cell factor which regulate the proliferation of haemopoietic progenitor cells. Br J Haematol 1996;94:606–611.

14 Okuyama R, Koguma M, Yanai N, Obinata M: Bone marrow stromal cells induce myeloid and lymphoid development of the sorted hematopoietic stem cells in vitro. Blood 1995;86: 2590–2597.

15 Broudy VC, Kovach NL, Bennett LG, Lin N, Jacobsen FW, Kidd PG: Human umbilical vein endothelial cells display high-affinity c-kit receptors and produce a soluble form of the c-kit receptor. Blood 1994;83:2145–2152.
16 Lenhoff S, Olofsson T: Cytokine regulation of GM-CSF and G-CSF secretion by human umbilical cord vein endothelial cells (HUVEC). Cytokine 1996;8:702–709.
17 Kobayashi H: Effect of c-kit ligand (stem cell factor) in combination with interleukin-5, granulocyte-macrophage colony-stimulating factor, and interleukin-3 on eosinophil lineage. Int J Hematol 1993;58:21–26.
18 Ichihara M, Hotta T, Asano H, Inoue C, Murate T, Kobayashi M, Saito H: Effects of stem cell factor (SCF) on human marrow neutrophil, neutrophil/macrophage mixed, macrophage and eosinophil progenitor cell growth. Int J Hematol 1994;59:81–89.
19 Kaplanski G, Teysseire N, Farnarier C, Kaplanski S, Lissitzky JC, Durand JM, Soubeyrand J, Dinarello CA, Bongrand P: IL-6 and IL-8 production from cultured human endothelial cells stimulated by interferon with *Rickettsia conorii* via a cell-associated IL-1α-dependent pathway. J Clin Invest 1995;96:2839–2844.
20 Fabian I, Lass M, Kletter Y, Golde DW: Differentiation and functional activity of human eosinophilic cells from an eosinophil HL-60 subline: Response to recombinant hematopoietic growth factors. Blood 1992;80:788–794.
21 Elsas MI, Elsas PX, Joseph D, Havet N, Da Silva LA, Salgado DR, Saliou B, Vargaftig BB: Stimulation of early eosinophil progenitors by a heat stable alveolar macrophage product from ovalbumin-sensitized and non-sensitized guinea pigs. Clin Exp Allergy 1997;27:208–217.
22 Lenhoff S, Olofsson T: Cytokine regulation of GM-CSF and G-CSF secretion by human umbilical cord vein endothelial cells (HUVEC). Cytokine 1996;8:702–709.
23 Ema H, Suda T, Nagayoshi K, Miura Y, Civin CI, Nakauchi H: Target cells for granulocyte colony-stimulating factor, interleukin-3, and interleukin-5 in differentiation pathway of neutrophils and eosinophils. Blood 1990;76:1956–1961.

International Archives of
Allergy and
Immunology

Int Arch Allergy Immunol 1999;120(suppl 1):7–10

Ecalectin as a T Cell-Derived Eosinophil Chemoattractant

Mitsuomi Hirashima

Department of Immunology and Immunopathology, Kagawa Medical School, Kagawa, Japan

Key Words
Eosinophil · Ecalectin · Galectin · Chemotaxis · T cell

Abstract
In our previous papers, we have shown that human T cells produce a unique eosinophil chemotactic factor (ECF), termed Ecalectin, with a molecular weight of about 30–50 kD during interaction with BALL-1 (a B cell line) extracts, antigen or mitogen. A 1.6-kB cDNA was isolated from a human T cell-derived expression library that encodes Ecalectin. Ecalectin is a 36-kD protein consisting of 323 amino acids based on its deduced amino acid sequence. Ecalectin was found to be a variant of human galectin-9, a member of the growing family of animal lectins exhibiting affinity for β-galactosides. Recombinant Ecalectin, expressed in COS cells, exhibited potent ECF activity in vitro and in vivo in a dose-dependent manner but not chemotactic activity for neutrophils, lymphocytes, or monocytes. The finding that the Ecalectin transcript is present in various lymphatic tissues and that its expression increases substantially in antigen-activated peripheral blood mononuclear cells suggests that Ecalectin is an important T cell-derived regulator of eosinophil recruitment in allergic reaction sites.

Introduction

Eosinophils play a central role in pathological conditions such as allergic inflammation, helminth infections, and even cancer, which are characterized by the accumulation of eosinophils in tissues (i.e. tissue eosinophilia) governed by the presence of eosinophil chemotactic factors (ECF). A variety of ECF have been identified. These include: (1) lipid inflammatory mediators, such as platelet-derived factor and 5-lipoxygenase metabolites of arachidonic acid, (2) complement fragments C3a and C5a, (3) cytokines, such as interleukin-3 (IL-3), IL-5 and granulocyte-macrophage colony-stimulating factor (GM-CSF), and (4) chemokines of the C-C family, which includes RANTES, MIP-1α, MCP-1, MCP-2, MCP-3, MCP-4 and eotaxin. Various types of cells, such as mast cells, monocytes/macrophages, and lymphocytes, can produce ECFs [1]. For example, the conditioned medium collected from antigen-stimulated T lymphocytes was shown to be chemotactic for eosinophils suggesting that T cells can produce ECF [2–4]. Even though IL-3, IL-5 and GM-CSF can be produced by T cells, we have previously shown that the ECF activity induced by the conditioned medium of antigen-stimulated T cells is not due to these cytokines [5, 6]. In this review, we discuss the evidence for the involvement of T cell-derived ECF in human diseases, and we propose that the newly isolated T cell-derived ECF called Ecalectin plays a crucial role in the specific recruitment of eosinophils.

KARGER
Fax + 41 61 306 12 34
E-Mail karger@karger.ch
www.karger.com

1018–2438/99/1205–0007$17.50/0

Accessible online at:
http://BioMedNet.com/karger

Dr. Mitsuomi Hirashima
Department of Immunology and Immunopathology
Kagawa Medical School, 1750-1 Ikenobe, Miki-cho
Kita-gun, Kagawa 761-0793 (Japan)
Tel. +81 87 891 2117, Fax +81 87 891 2119, E-Mail mitsuomi@kms.ac.jp

T Cell-Derived ECF in Humans

It is well known that the allergic inflammatory response, such as bronchial asthma, is divided into two phases: the immediate phase, which occurs within 30 min, and the late phase, which peaks 6 h after antigenic challenge. Similarly, the phenomenon of tissue eosinophilia is characterized by two phases, namely the early and delayed phases, which occur 6 h and 24 h after antigenic challenge, respectively [7]. What are the ECF involved during these two phases? Previous studies have demonstrated that C-C chemokines may be responsible for the recruitment of eosinophils during the early phase of tissue eosinophilia, since mRNA levels of RANTES and eotaxin were found to be elevated in lesions during this phase [8]. However, other ECF appear to be important during the delayed phase of tissue eosinophilia. Indeed, there is evidence to suggest that the newly isolated ECF, Ecalectin (40–60 kD), is involved. Ecalectin was first isolated from the guinea pig model of tissue eosinophilia during the delayed phase [7], and was found to be mainly produced by antigen-specific T cells [3, 9]. A similar T cell-derived ECF, which corresponds to the Ecalectin in the guinea pig has also been isolated in humans [4–6].

In our laboratory, we have been interested in the study of T cell-derived ECF in cancer, and a result of these studies led to the isolation of human Ecalectin. First, peripheral blood mononuclear cells (PBMC) were cultured with irradiated B cells of the BALL-1 cell line, and we found that an ECF of 30–50 kD was largely produced [10, 11]. So, in order to test whether the proliferation of T cells, occurring following their interaction with BALL-1 extracts, was sufficient to induce the production of ECF, T cells were stimulated with the T cell growth factor, IL-2. Using a Rotofor system, the isoelectric point (PI) of the ECF produced by IL-2- and BALL-1-stimulated T cells was assayed, and was found to be at pH 5 and 7, respectively. This difference of PI suggested that the proliferation of T cells is not sufficient to induce the production of the BALL-1-dependent ECF (B1-ECF), and that other mechanisms must be involved. Indeed, the production of the B1-ECF appeared to be dependent on specific interactions between PBMC and BALL-1 cells, since no ECF activity was obtained when PBMC were cultured with extracts of other B cell lines, such as Daudi, Nalm-1, and Namalwa [10]. Further studies suggest that an unknown glycoprotein found in the plasma membrane of BALL-1 cells might be responsible for the production of B1-ECF by T cells [11].

Other non-ECF biological functions of the B1-ECF were also examined. For example, its effect on the respiratory burst of eosinophils was studied. We found that B1-ECF strongly suppressed superoxide release from eosinophils stimulated with fMLP [5, 10]. Interestingly, these results were in contrast to those obtained with the ECF produced by IL-2-stimulated T cells (IL-2-ECF). In this case, IL-2-ECF enhanced the release of superoxide from eosinophils, contributing to the evidence that B1-ECF differs from IL-2-ECF.

Cloning and Characterization of Human Ecalectin

In the process of cloning human Ecalectin, we generated a T cell line which constitutively produced B1-ECF by transforming STO-2 cells using the HTLV-1 virus system [6]. STO-2-derived Ecalectin, or human native Ecalectin was purified by isoelectric electrophoresis using a Rotofor system and by gel filtration using a Superose 12 column [12]. In order to generate antibodies against Ecalectin, human native Ecalectin was injected into rabbits. Following their purification, anti-Ecalectin antibodies were used for the cloning of the Ecalectin gene from the cDNA library of STO-2-transformed cells [12]. Recombinant human Ecalectin was also generated by transfecting COS cells with the cloned cDNA of Ecalectin [12], and its PI was assayed. Although native Ecalectin has a PI of pH 7, the PI of recombinant human Ecalectin derived from COS cells was found to be around pH 8. The reason for and the significance of this difference in PI is presently unknown.

Human native Ecalectin was found to be a 36-kD protein of 323 amino acids which shares high homology (98%) with one of the 10 members of the galectin family, galectin-9 [12]. Like galectins, Ecalectin was found to have binding affinity for lactose, since most of the Ecalectin-induced ECF activity is generated when using the eluted fraction obtained from a lactose column. Moreover, three sites of N-glycosylation (positions 34, 79 and 137) have been found on human native Ecalectin, which are different from the positions of the glycosylated sites found in murine Ecalectin [13]. Many tissues were shown to express Ecalectin. In the case of lymphoid tissues, Ecalectin was highly expressed in the spleen and in lymph nodes. Furthermore, we have found that the thymus, the bone marrow, and the fetal liver express comparable levels of Ecalectin transcripts [12]. The presence of Ecalectin mRNA was also detected in nonlymphoid organs, such as the lung, the intestine and the stomach [12]. It is not surprising that Ecalectin is expressed in these organs, since tissue eosinophilia has been shown to occur in these sites [13].

Regulation of Ecalectin Production

As in the case of Ecalectin from the guinea pig, there is evidence to suggest that the production of the human Ecalectin requires antigen stimulation. For example, it was shown that Ecalectin levels increased by 50- to 90-fold in PBMC isolated from patients with *Dermatofagoides farinae* (Df) when they were stimulated with the antigen (Df) for a period of 48 h; PBMC left unstimulated expressed low levels of Ecalectin mRNA [12]. Similar results were also obtained when Ecalectin protein levels were assayed by SDS-PAGE/immunoblot analysis. Only antigen-stimulated cells expressed high levels of Ecalectin protein [12].

In the guinea pig model, the production of Ecalectin by antigen-stimulated T cells is potentiated by an ECF-potentiating factor (ECF-PF) of 10–20 kD produced by macrophages [9]. The production of human Ecalectin appears to involve a similar mechanism [14, 15]. For example, it was shown that PBMC obtained from tuberculin-sensitive patients, and restimulated in vitro with the antigen (PPD), produced little ECF since very low levels of ECF activity were obtained [13]. However, if tuberculin-sensitive PBMC were pretreated with IL-4 or with an ECF-PF obtained from macrophages treated with lipopolysaccharide, the production of the 40- to 60-kD ECF, now known to be Ecalectin, was greatly enhanced [14, 15]. Surprisingly, the production of IL-5 by tuberculin-sensitive PBMC was suppressed following IL-4 treatment [15].

Biological Properties of Ecalectin

Recombinant Ecalectin produced by Ecalectin-positive COS cells is a potent ECF. Indeed, the recombinant Ecalectin-induced ECF activity was found to be much greater than that of RANTES and IL-5, and almost reached that of eotaxin [12]. In vitro, the chemotaxis-inducing activity of Ecalectin was shown to be selective for eosinophils, since it had no effect on the chemotaxis of neutrophils, monocytes and lymphocytes [12]. Furthermore, the ECF activity of Ecalectin was also demonstrated in vivo. Indeed, when Ecalectin was injected into the peritoneal cavity of mice, it was found that eosinophils selectively accumulated at the site of injection [12].

Ecalectin has biological functions other than its ECF activity. Using native Ecalectin, we found that it can enhance the surface expression of Fcε and Fcγ receptors, and suppress the release of superoxide from eosinophils [5, 6, 10]. Moreover, results obtained from preliminary experiments using flow cytometry to assess hydrogen peroxide (H_2O_2) release indicated that Ecalectin has a suppressive effect on H_2O_2 release of PMA-treated eosinophils. Finally, there is evidence to suggest that Ecalectin is implicated in the apoptotic death of eosinophils. Recent experiments demonstrated that dexamethasone-induced apoptosis of eosinophils was significantly attenuated by the treatment with Ecalectin.

Interestingly, another study demonstrated that murine galectin-9 can cause the apoptosis of thymocytes and activated T cells, suggesting that Ecalectin may have an effect on the apoptosis of these cells [16, 17].

Conclusion

In summary, a new T cell-derived ECF has been described which has been called Ecalectin. The production of Ecalectin T cells requires antigenic stimulation, and this is potentiated by a macrophage-derived ECF-PF. The Ecalectin gene was found to be homologous to the galectin-9 gene, and this homology to galectin-9 is of pathological relevance since galectin-9 is thought to play a role in Hodgkin's disease (HD). Indeed, galectin-9 was first cloned from the lymph node of patients with HD, and 50% of patients with HD were found to have antibodies against galectin-9 in their serum [18]. Moreover, it is well known that patients with a particular form of HD (mixed cellularity HD) exhibit marked tissue eosinophilia in their lymph nodes. Furthermore, a study by Kay et al. [19] demonstrated that ECF activity is generated from the lymph node cells of HD patients. Thus, it is likely that Ecalectin also plays a role in the pathogenesis of HD. Finally, because galectin-9 can induce the apoptosis of thymocytes in the murine system [17], it would be of great interest to investigate whether Ecalectin can also induce apoptosis of thymocytes in humans, and thus contribute to the process of T cell maturation.

Acknowledgements

We thank Sophie Chabot (PhD graduate student/University of Calgary) for her critical reading of the manuscript.

References

1 Hirashima M: Eosinophil chemotactic factors; in Makino S, Fukuda T (eds): Eosinophils; Biological and Clinical Aspects. Boca Raton, CRC Press, 1993, pp 227–240.

2 Hirotsu Y, Hirashima M, Hayashi H: The mediation of tissue eosinophilia in hypersensitivity reactions. III. Separation of two different eosinophil chemotactic factors and transfer of those factors by serum or cells from sensitized guinea pigs. Immunology 1983;48:59–67.

3 Hirashima M, Hirotsu Y, Hayashi H: The mediation of tissue eosinophilia in hypersensitivity reactions. IV. Production of delayed eosinophil chemotactic factor-a by peritoneal exudate cells from sensitized guinea pigs in vitro. Immunology 1983;48:69–77.

4 Hirashima M, Okooronkwo MO, Takahashi T, Takamura S, Tono-oka S: Involvement of monocytes in preferential production of eosinophil chemotactic lymphokine in patients with schistosomiasis. Kumamoto Med J 1990;42: 33–44.

5 Hirashima M, Ueno M, Kamiya K, Higuchi S, Matsumoto R: Functional heterogeneity of human eosinophil chemotactic lymphokines. Lymphokine Cytokine Res 1991;10:481–486.

6 Hirashima M, Ueno M, Higuchi S, Matsumoto T, Sakata K, Matsumoto R, Adachi M: Establishment of a human T-cell line constitutively producing chemotactic lymphokines and their heterogeneity on eosinophils. Lymphokine Cytokine Res 1992;11:331–338.

7 Hirashima M, Hayashi H: The mediation of tissue eosinophilia in hypersensitivity reactions. I. Isolation of two different chemotactic factors from DNP-ascaris extract-induced skin lesions in guinea pigs. Immunology 1976;30: 203–212.

8 Rothenberg ME, Luster AD, Lilly CM, Drazen JM, Leder P: Constitutive and allergen-induced expression of eotaxin mRNA in the guinea pig lung. J Exp Med 1995;181:1211–1216.

9 Sakata K-M, Tashiro K, Hirashima M, Hayashi H: Selective regulation of chemotactic lymphokine production. I. Selective potentiation of eosinophil chemotactic lymphokine production in the alum hydroxy gel- and *Bordetella pertussis* vaccine-treated guinea pigs. J Immunol 1985;133:3463–3467.

10 Hirashima M, Ueno M, Saita N, Takamura S, Watanabe K, Tsurufuji S, Adachi M: Induction of an eosinophil chemotactic factor production from T lymphocytes by a B cell lymphoma line. Immunol Lett 1993;36:273–281.

11 Seki M, Hirashima M: Induction of eosinophil chemotactic factor production from human peripheral blood mononuclear cells by solubilized BALL-1, a B-cell lymphoma line. Int Arch Allergy Immunol 1997;114:2–5.

12 Matsumoto R, Matsumoto H, Seki M, Hata M, Asano Y, Kanegasaki S, Stevens RL, Hirashima M: Human ecalectin, a variant human galectin-9, is a novel chemoattractant produced by T lymphocytes. J Biol Chem 1998;273: 16976–16984.

13 Spry CJF: Eosinophils: A comprehensive Review and Guide to the Scientific and Medical Literature. Oxford, Oxford University Press, 1989.

14 Hata T, Hirashima M: Effects of IL-4 on antigen-induced production of eosinophil chemotactic activity from human mononuclear leukocytes. Int Arch Allergy Immunol 1997;114: 6–9.

15 Nishiyama T, Hata T, Okada H, Hirashima M: Short-term stimulation with interleukin-4 enhances PPD-induced production of an eosinophil chemotactic lymphokine but suppresses IL-5 production. Allergol Int 1998;47:37–43.

16 Wada J, Kanwar YS: Identification and characterization of galectin-9, a novel beta-galactoside-binding mammalian lectin. J Biol Chem 1997;272:6078–6086.

17 Wada J, Ota K, Kumar A, Wallner EI, Kanwar YS: Developmental regulation, expression, and apoptotic potential of galectin-9, a beta-galactoside binding lectin. J Clin Invest 1997;99: 2452–2461.

18 Tureci O, Schmit H, Fadel N, Pfreundschuh M, Sahin U: Molecular definition of a novel human galectin which is immunogenic in patients with Hodgkin's disease. J Biol Chem 1997;272:6416–6422.

19 Kay AB, McVie JG, Stuart AE, Krajewski A, Turnbull LW: Eosinophil chemotaxis of supernatants from cultured Hodgkin's lymph node cells. J Clin Pathol 1975;28:502–505.

International Archives of
Allergy and Immunology

Int Arch Allergy Immunol 1999;120(suppl 1):11–14

Analysis of Biological Activities of Recombinant Rat Interleukin-5

Kenji Ishihara Takeaki Nittoh Ikuko Satoh Kazuo Ohuchi

Department of Pathophysiological Biochemistry, Graduate School of Pharmaceutical Sciences, Tohoku University, Miyagi, Japan

Key Words
Interleukin-5 · B cell growth factor II · Eosinophil differentiation factor · Eosinophil survival-enhancing factor

Abstract
We analyzed the biological activities of recombinant rat interleukin-5 (IL-5). Purified recombinant rat IL-5 promoted the proliferation of T88-M cells in a concentration-dependent manner, and its effect was inhibited by an anti-murine IL-5-neutralizing polyclonal antibody. When bone marrow cells from normal rats were incubated with recombinant rat IL-5 in medium containing methylcellulose, the colony formation by eosinophilic cells was induced. Furthermore, when rat peritoneal eosinophils were incubated with recombinant rat IL-5, the spontaneous decrease in eosinophil viability was inhibited in a time- and concentration-dependent manner. In addition, the recombinant rat IL-5-induced eosinophil survival was inhibited by an anti-murine IL-5-neutralizing polyclonal antibody. These findings suggest that rat IL-5 acts as B cell growth factor II, eosinophil differentiation factor, and eosinophil survival-enhancing factor.

Introduction

Gene cloning of human and mouse interleukin-5 (IL-5) and preparation of their recombinant IL-5 have promoted the analysis of the roles of IL-5 in allergic inflammation, especially in eosinophil function, in both species [1–5]. In rats, although it was suggested that IL-5 plays a significant role in eosinophil function in allergic inflammation [6–9], direct evidence showing the role of rat IL-5 in eosinophil function has not been obtained because recombinant rat IL-5 was not available. Recently, we have prepared recombinant rat IL-5 by a baculovirus expression system using cDNA for rat IL-5 [10]. The present paper describes the biological activities of recombinant rat IL-5 and compares the activity with that of human and mouse IL-5.

Materials and Methods

Preparation of Recombinant Rat IL-5
Recombinant rat IL-5 was expressed in silkworm *Bombyx mori* larvae and purified by anion exchange chromatography and hydrophobic chromatography. The final purification of recombinant rat IL-5 was more than 95.5%. The details for the preparation of recombinant rat IL-5 are described elsewhere [10].

Cell Growth Assay
T88-M cells [11, 12] obtained from RIKEN Gene Bank (Tsukuba, Japan) were used for the determination of IL-5 activity which was

KARGER
Fax +41 61 306 12 34
E-Mail karger@karger.ch
www.karger.com

1018–2438/99/1205–0011$17.50/0

Accessible online at:
http://BioMedNet.com/karger

Kazuo Ohuchi, PhD
Department of Pathophysiological Biochemistry
Graduate School of Pharmaceutical Sciences, Tohoku University
Aoba Aramaki, Aoba-ku, Sendai, Miyagi 980-8578 (Japan)
Tel. +81 22 217 6860, Fax +81 22 217 6859, E-Mail ohuchi-k@mail.pharm.tohoku.ac.jp

assessed by a modification of the cell growth assay described by Kobayashi et al. [13]. T88-M cells were seeded in each well of 96-well plates at a density of 1 × 10^4 cells in 0.1 ml of RPMI-1640 medium (Gibco BRL, Gaithersburg, Md., USA) supplemented with 1% (v/v) fetal bovine serum (FBS; Flow Laboratories, North Rydge, Australia) containing various concentrations of recombinant rat IL-5 in the presence or absence of an anti-murine IL-5-neutralizing polyclonal antibody (R & D Systems, Minneapolis, Minn., USA), and incubated for 48 h at 37 °C. The cells were pulse-labeled with 5 µl/well of MTT (3-[4,5-dimethylthiazol-2-yl]-2,5-diphenyltetrazolium bromide; Sigma Chemical Co.) solution (5 mg/ml in PBS) for the last 4 h of culture. After the removal of 70 µl of medium, MTT products were dissolved with 100 µl of dimethylsulfoxide, and the absorbance at 570 nm relative to 630 nm was measured with a microplate reader.

Colony Formation

Colony formation was performed by a modification of the methylcellulose culture method described by Yamaguchi et al. [14]. Bone marrow cells collected from shinbones and thighbones of normal rats were seeded in each well of 6-well plates at a density of 4 × 10^4 cells in 4 ml of 1.2% (w/v) methylcellulose (Wako Pure Chemical Industries, Osaka, Japan) αMEM (Gibco BRL) supplemented with 30% (v/v) FBS and 1% (w/v) bovine serum albumin (BSA; Sigma Chemical Co.) in the presence or absence of 100 p*M* recombinant rat IL-5, and incubated for 6 days. The number of colonies was counted and each colony was suspended in medium containing 30% (v/v) FBS and 1% (w/v) BSA. The cells in each colony were identified after May-Grünwald-Giemsa staining.

Determination of Survival of Rat Eosinophils

Rat peritoneal eosinophils were prepared according to our previous report [15]. The purity of eosinophils was more than 95% as assessed by May-Grünwald-Giemsa staining, and the viability of eosinophils was more than 98% by the trypan blue exclusion test. The purified peritoneal eosinophils were seeded in each well of 96-well plates at a density of 1 × 10^5 cells in 0.1 ml of RPMI-1640 medium supplemented with 10% (v/v) FBS containing various concentrations of recombinant rat IL-5 in the presence or absence of an anti-murine IL-5-neutralizing polyclonal antibody and incubated at 37 °C for the periods indicated. After incubation, the viability of eosinophils was determined by the ability to exclude trypan blue dye. The viability of eosinophils was calculated from the following equation: viability (%) = (number of cells that excluded trypan blue/number of total cells) × 100.

Statistical Analysis

The statistical significance of the results was analyzed by Dunnett's test for multiple comparison.

Results and Discussion

BCGF-II Activity of Recombinant Rat IL-5 in T88-M Cells

Überla et al. [16] reported that T88-M cells and B13 cells, IL-5-dependent mouse B cell lines, were proliferated by transfection of rat IL-5 gene or by incubation with the supernatant of rat IL-5 gene-transfected T88-M cells or B13 cells. However, they failed to show direct effects of recombinant rat IL-5 because they did not isolate it. We therefore examined whether recombinant rat IL-5 directly promotes proliferation of T88-M cells. A significant increase in the proliferation of T88-M cells was induced by recombinant rat IL-5 in a concentration-dependent manner at 0.1–100 p*M* when determined by MTT assay 48 h after incubation (table 1). The proliferation of T88-M cells by recombinant rat IL-5 was inhibited by an anti-murine IL-5-neutralizing polyclonal antibody in a concentration-dependent manner (table 1). These findings strongly indicate that recombinant rat IL-5 possesses B cell growth factor II (BCGF-II) activity.

Table 1. Effects of recombinant rat IL-5 on proliferation of T88-M cells

Rat IL-5 p*M*	Anti-mIL-5 pAb ng/ml	Proliferation % of control
0	0	$100.0 \pm 4.9^{\#\#\#}$
0.1	0	$195.1 \pm 8.1^{***, \#\#\#}$
1	0	$232.4 \pm 7.1^{***, \#\#\#}$
10	0	$437.3 \pm 11.1^{***, \#\#\#}$
100	0	$685.3 \pm 11.0^{***}$
100	100	$401.0 \pm 19.1^{***, \#\#\#}$
100	1,000	$264.7 \pm 23.4^{***, \#\#\#}$

Values are the means ± SEM from 6 samples. See Materials and Methods for procedure. *** $p < 0.001$ vs. 0 p*M* rat IL-5; ### $p < 0.001$ vs. 100 p*M* rat IL-5.

Table 2. Effects of recombinant rat IL-5 on colony formation by bone marrow cells from normal rats

Rat IL-5 p*M*	Total colonies	Eosinophilic colonies	Eosinophilic colonies, %
0	0	0	0
100	17	17	100

See Materials and Methods for specifications. The results were confirmed by another set of experiments.

Effects of Recombinant Rat IL-5 on Rat Eosinophils

IL-5 induces differentiation and proliferation of bone marrow cells to eosinophils [14] and maintains eosinophil survival [17, 18] in humans and mice. An increase in the number of eosinophils is regarded to be a trigger of pathogenesis of allergic inflammation such as asthma and atopic dermatitis [5, 19–21]. In rats, although a possible participation of eosinophils in allergic inflammation has been studied [6–9, 15], it has not been clarified whether rat IL-5 regulates the function of rat eosinophils. Therefore, we assessed whether recombinant rat IL-5 possesses eosinophil differentiation factor (EDF) activity and eosinophil survival-enhancing activity. EDF activity was determined by colony formation of bone marrow cells from normal rats using the methylcellulose culture method. After 6 days of culture, colony formation was observed when the rat bone marrow cells were incubated in the presence of 100 p*M* recombinant rat IL-5, but not in the absence of IL-5 (table 2). Staining of each colony by May-Grünwald-Giemsa revealed that all of these colonies were formed by eosinophils (table 2). These findings indicate that recombinant rat IL-5 possesses EDF activity. Furthermore, we assessed eosinophil survival-enhancing activity of recombinant rat IL-5. When rat eosinophils were incubated at 37 °C, the viability of the cells decreased time-dependently (fig. 1a). A significant decrease in viability was observed at 48, 72, and 96 h (fig. 1a). In contrast, when incubated in the presence of recombinant rat IL-5 at 100 p*M*, the viability of eosinophils was maintained for up to 96 h (fig. 1a). The viability of eosinophils incubated in the presence of recombinant rat IL-5 was significantly higher than that of control eosinophils at 24, 48, 72, and 96 h (fig. 1a). Recombinant rat IL-5 prolonged the survival of rat eosinophils in a concentration-dependent manner at 1–100 p*M* when examined 96 h after incubation (fig. 1b). The prolongation of the survival of rat eosinophils by recombinant rat IL-5 at 100 p*M* was inhibited by an anti-murine IL-5-neutralizing polyclonal antibody in a concentration-dependent manner (fig. 1c). These findings indicate that recombinant rat IL-5 possesses eosinophil survival-enhancing activity.

In conclusion, we found that recombinant rat IL-5 shows BCGF-II activity, EDF activity, and eosinophil survival-enhancing activity. Recombinant rat IL-5 will contribute to analyze the role of eosinophils in allergic inflammation in rats.

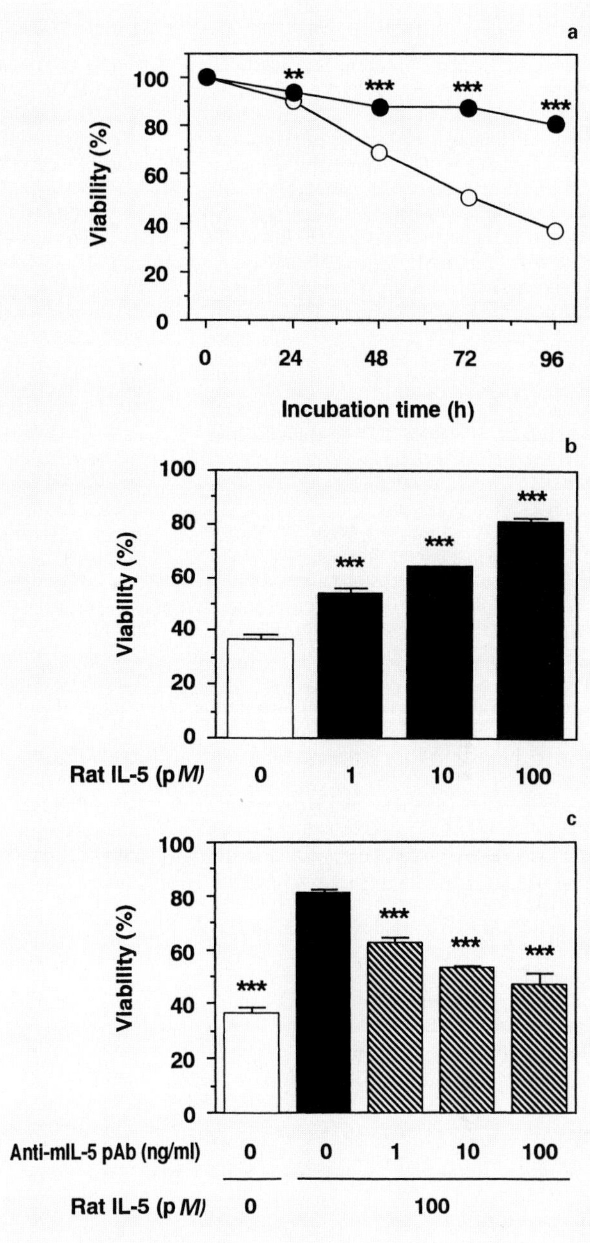

Fig. 1. Effects of recombinant rat IL-5 on the viability of rat eosinophils. **a** 1 × 10^5 cells were incubated at 37 °C for the periods indicated in 0.1 ml of RPMI-1640 medium supplemented with 10% (v/v) FBS in the presence (●) or absence (○) of 100 p*M* recombinant rat IL-5. **b** 1 × 10^5 cells were incubated for 96 h at 37 °C in 0.1 ml of RPMI-1640 medium supplemented with 10% (v/v) FBS containing the indicated concentrations of recombinant rat IL-5 or (**c**) anti-murine IL-5-neutralizing polyclonal antibody (anti-mIL-5 pAb) in the presence of 100 p*M* recombinant rat IL-5. The viability of eosinophils was determined by the ability to exclude trypan blue dye. Values are means ± SEM from 5 samples shown by vertical bars. In **a**, SEM is within each circle. **a** ** $p < 0.01$, *** $p < 0.001$ vs. corresponding control; **b** *** $p < 0.001$ vs. 0 p*M* rat IL-5; **c** *** $p < 0.001$ vs. 100 p*M* rat IL-5 without anti-mIL-5 pAb.

Acknowledgments

We are grateful to Prof. Akira Tominaga, Kochi Medical School, Nangoku, Kochi, Japan, for providing us with T88-M cells. B151K12 cells were a gift from Prof. Kiyoshi Takatsu, Institute of Medical Science, University of Tokyo, Tokyo, Japan.

References

1 Azuma C, Tanabe T, Konishi M, Kinashi T, Noma T, Matsuda F, Yaoita Y, Takatsu K, Hammarström L, Smith CIE, Severinson E, Honjo T: Cloning of cDNA for human T-cell replacing factor (interleukin-5) and comparison with the murine homologue. Nucleic Acids Res 1986;14:9149–9158.

2 Kinashi T, Harada N, Severinson E, Tanabe T, Sideras P, Konishi M, Azuma C, Tominaga A, Bergstedt-Lindqvist S, Takahashi M, Matsuda F, Yaoita Y, Takatsu K, Honjo T: Cloning of complementary DNA encoding T-cell replacing factor and identity with B-cell growth factor II. Nature 1986;324:70–73.

3 Proudfoot AEI, Fattah D, Kawashima EH, Bernard A, Wingfield PT: Preparation and characterization of human interleukin-5 expressed in recombinant *Escherichia coli*. Biochem J 1990;270:357–361.

4 Kunimoto DY, Allison KC, Watson C, Fuerst T, Armstrong GD, Paul W, Strober W: High-level production of murine interleukin-5 (IL-5) utilizing recombinant baculovirus expression. Purification of the rIL-5 and its use assessing the biologic role of IL-5 glycosylation. Cytokine 1991;3:224–230.

5 Koike M, Takatsu K: IL-5 and its receptor: Which role do they play in the immune response? Int Arch Allergy Immunol 1994;104:1-9.

6 Kitagaki K, Niwa S, Hoshiko K, Nagai H, Hayashi S, Totsuka T: Augmentation of apoptosis in bronchial exuded rat eosinophils by cyclosporin A. Biochem Biophys Res Commun 1996;222:71–77.

7 Haczku A, Macary P, Haddad E-B, Huang TJ, Kemeny DM, Moqbel R, Chung KF: Expression of Th-2 cytokines interleukin-4 and -5 and of Th-1 cytokine interferon-γ in ovalbumin-exposed sensitized Brown-Norway rats. Immunology 1996;88:247–251.

8 Nittoh T, Arii M, Suzuki R, Kitoh A, Watanabe M, Mue S, Ohuchi K: Increase in eosinophilic cell population in bone marrow of rats by immunization with *Ascaris suum* antigen. Immunol Invest 1997;26:439–451.

9 Underwood SL, Raeburn D, Lawrence C, Foster M, Webber S, Karlsson J-A: RPR 106541, a novel, airways-selective glucocorticoid: Effects against antigen-induced CD4+T lymphocyte accumulation and cytokine gene expression in the Brown Norway rat lung. Brit J Pharmacol 1997;122:439–446.

10 Ishihara K, Satoh I, Nittoh T, Kanaya T, Okazaki H, Suzuki T, Koyama T, Sakamoto T, Ide T, Ohuchi K: Preparation of recombinant rat interleukin-5 by baculovirus expression system and analysis of its biological activities. Biochim Biophys Acta 1999; in press.

11 Mita S, Tominaga A, Hitoshi Y, Sakamoto K, Honjo T, Akagi M, Kikuchi Y, Yamaguchi N, Takatsu K: Characterization of high-affinity receptors for interleukin 5 on interleukin 5-dependent cell lines. Proc Natl Acad Sci USA 1989;86:2311–2315.

12 Tominaga A, Mita S, Kikuchi Y, Hitoshi Y, Takatsu K, Nishikawa S, Ogawa M: Establishment of IL-5-dependent early B cell lines by long-term bone marrow cultures. Growth Factors 1989;1:135–146.

13 Kobayashi Y, Saheki T, Shinozawa T: Induction of PC12 cell death, apoptosis, by a sialoglycopeptide from bovine brain. Biochem Biophys Res Commun 1994;203:1554–1559.

14 Yamaguchi Y, Suda T, Suda J, Eguchi M, Miura Y, Harada N, Tominaga A, Takatsu K: Purified interleukin 5 supports the terminal differentiation and proliferation of murine eosinophilic precursors. J Exp Med 1988;167:43–56.

15 Watanabe M, Nittoh T, Suzuki T, Kitoh A, Mue S, Ohuchi K: Isolation and partial characterization of eosinophil granule proteins in rats – Eosinophil cationic protein and major basic protein. Int Arch Allergy Immunol 1995;108:11–18.

16 Überla K, Li W, Qin Z, Richter G, Raabe T, Diamantstein T, Blankenstein T: The rat interleukin-5 gene: Characterization and expression by retroviral gene transfer and polymerase chain reaction. Cytokine 1991;3:72–81.

17 Yamaguchi Y, Hayashi Y, Sugama Y, Miura Y, Kasahara T, Kitamura S, Torisu M, Mita S, Tominaga A, Takatsu K, Suda T: Highly purified murine interleukin 5 (IL-5) stimulates eosinophil function and prolongs in vitro survival. IL-5 as an eosinophil chemotactic factor. J Exp Med 1988;167:1737–1742.

18 Yamaguchi Y, Suda T, Ohta S, Tominaga K, Miura Y, Kasahara T: Analysis of the survival of mature human eosinophils: Interleukin-5 prevents apoptosis in mature human eosinophils. Blood 1991;78:2542–2547.

19 Bousquet J, Chanez P, Lacoste JY, Barnéon G, Ghanavian N, Enander I, Venge P, Ahlstedt S, Simony-Lafontaine J, Godard P, Michel F-B: Eosinophilic inflammation in asthma. N Engl J Med 1990;323:1033–1039.

20 Corrigan CJ, Kay AB: T cells and eosinophils in the pathogenesis of asthma. Immunol Today 1992;13:501–507.

21 Leung DYM: Atopic dermatitis: The skin as a window into the pathogenesis of chronic allergic disease. J Allergy Clin Immunol 1995;96:302–319.

International Archives of Allergy and Immunology

Int Arch Allergy Immunol 1999;120(suppl 1):15–18

Primary Role of CD4+ T Cells and Supplemental Role of Mast Cells in Allergic Pulmonary Eosinophilia

Koji Ogawa[a,b] Osamu Kaminuma[a,b] Hideo Kikkawa[b] Rieko Kameda[b] Katsuo Ikezawa[b] Matsunobu Suko[a] Hirokazu Okudaira[a] Kazuo Akiyama[c] Akio Mori[a,c]

[a]Department of Medicine and Physical Therapy, Faculty of Medicine, University of Tokyo, [b]Discovery Research Laboratory, Tanabe Seiyaku Co., Toda, Saitama, and [c]Clinical Research Center, National Sagamihara Hospital, Sagamihara, Kanagawa, Japan

Key Words

CD4+ T cell · Mast cell · Eosinophil · IL-5 · Mouse

Abstract

Background: We have recently demonstrated that allergic eosinophilic inflammation is transferred to unprimed mice by infusing IL-5-producing CD4+ T cells. The contribution of mast cells to the development of eosinophilic inflammation is controversial. ***Methods:*** To clarify the possible different roles of CD4+ T cells and mast cells in eosinophilic inflammation, we compared antigen-induced airway eosinophilia between mast-cell-deficient mice (WBB6F1-W/W^v) and their congenic normal littermates (WBB6F1-+/+). ***Results:*** The time course study indicated that equivalent numbers of eosinophils were recruited into the airway of both +/+ and W/W^v mice 6, 24, 96, and 216 h after antigen challenge, whereas the number of eosinophils 48 h after antigen challenge was significantly lower in W/W^v compared to +/+ mice. Administration of either anti-CD4 or anti-IL-5 monoclonal antibody almost completely inhibited antigen-induced eosinophil recruitment in W/W^v mice 48 h after antigen challenge. In contrast, the inhibitory effect of these antibodies in +/+ mice were partial (~50% inhibition). Anti-CD4 and anti-IL-5 antibodies equally suppressed airway eosinophilia in both +/+ and W/W^v mice 96 h after antigen challenge. ***Conclusion:*** Our study indicates that CD4+ T cells are crucially involved in the development of allergic eosinophilic inflammation, while mast cells may play a supplemental role depending on the kinetics of the response.

Introduction

Chronic eosinophilic inflammation of the bronchial mucosa is a prominent pathological feature of bronchial asthma [1]. Accumulating evidence suggests that IL-5 produced by activated CD4+ T cells play a central role in the local infiltration and activation of eosinophils [1, 2]. IL-5 production by peripheral blood T cells is markedly enhanced in both atopic and nonatopic asthmatics compared to healthy subjects [3, 4]. The development of eosinophilic inflammation in antigen-sensitized mice is dependent on CD4+ T cells and IL-5, since administration of antibodies against either CD4 or IL-5 significantly

KARGER

Fax + 41 61 306 12 34
E-Mail karger@karger.ch
www.karger.com

1018–2438/99/1205–0015$17.50/0

Accessible online at:
http://BioMedNet.com/karger

Dr. Koji Ogawa
Discovery Research Laboratory, Tanabe Seiyaku Co.
2-2-50 Kawagishi
Toda, Saitama 335-8505 (Japan)

reduced the induction of airway eosinophilia [5, 6]. In addition, we have recently demonstrated that the existence of IL-5-producing T cells is sufficient for the development of airway eosinophilic inflammation [7].

On the other hand, the involvement of mast cells in eosinophilic inflammation is still controversial. Mast cells secrete several cytokines, such as IL-3, IL-4, IL-5, IL-6, and tumor necrosis factor (TNF)-α in vitro, which can recruit, prime, and activate inflammatory cells including eosinophils [8–10]. Mast-cell-deficient mice, however, develop eosinophilic inflammation [11, 12], indicating that mast cells are not essential for the development of airway inflammatory responses.

In this study, we employed mast-cell-deficient mice and their congenic controls to demonstrate the primary role of CD4+ T cells in eosinophilic inflammation with a supplemental contribution by mast cells.

Materials and Methods

Materials

Male mast-cell-deficient mice (WBB6F1-W/W^v) and their congenic normal littermates (WBB6F1-+/+), 5 to 6 weeks of age, were obtained from Japan SLC (Shizuoka, Japan). Purified rat anti-mouse IL-5 monoclonal antibody (TRFK-5) was from Pharmingen (San Diego, Calif., USA), and ovalbumin (OVA) was from Sigma (St. Louis, Mo., USA). The hybridoma which generates rat anti-mouse CD4 monoclonal antibody (GK1.5) was obtained from ATCC (Rockville, Md., USA). GK1.5 was purified from ascitic fluid according to the procedure described previously [6].

Sensitization

Mice were sensitized by intraperitoneal injection of 0.2 ml antigen solution containing 200 μg OVA adsorbed to 6 mg aluminum hydroxide gel (alum). A booster injection of the alum/OVA mixture was given 14 days later.

Allergen Challenge

Fourteen days after the booster injection, mice were challenged with aerosolized OVA (100 mg/ml) dissolved in 0.9% saline delivered by a DeVilbiss 646 nebulizer (DeVilbiss, Somerset, Penn., USA) driven by compressed air at 18 liters/min for 20 min. As a control, 0.9% saline was administered by the same nebulizer. In some groups of animals, GK1.5 and TRFK-5 were injected intravenously, 6 days and 5 min before the antigen challenge, respectively. Fluorescence-activated cell sorter analysis of splenic cells confirmed that in vivo treatment with purified GK1.5 induced more than 90% depletion of the CD4+ population (data not shown).

Bronchoalveolar Lavage

Saline- or OVA-challenged mice were killed by excess intraperitoneal administration of sodium pentobarbital 6–216 h after antigen challenge. The trachea was cannulated with a polyethylene tube through which the lungs were gently lavaged with 0.5 ml Hank's balanced salt solution 4 times (2 ml total). The lavage fluid was then centrifuged at 1,500 rpm for 5 min. The pellet obtained was suspended in 250 μl Hank's balanced salt solution, and total cell number in BAL fluid (BALF) was counted by an automatic cell counter (Celltac MEK-5158; Nihon Kohden, Tokyo, Japan). Differential cell counts were made by microscopy of centrifuged preparations stained with May-Giemsa, counting 200 cells in each animal.

Statistics

All data are presented as means ± SEM. Statistical analysis was performed using Student's t test for comparison between two groups and one-way ANOVA and Bonferroni's method for 3 groups or more. Values of $p < 0.05$ were considered to be statistically significant.

Results and Discussion

The first experiment was carried out to compare the intensity of allergic airway eosinophilia between mast-cell-deficient mice and their congenic wild-type littermates. As shown in figure 1, airway eosinophilia observed in W/W^v mice 6, 24, 96 and 216 h after antigen challenge was not significantly different from that in +/+ mice, clearly indicating that mast cells are not essential for eosinophilic infiltration into the airway. Nevertheless, a significantly lower number of eosinophils was observed in BALF of W/W^v mice 48 h after challenge compared with +/+ mice, suggesting that mast cells contribute to airway eosinophilia at this time point. This difference in the eosinophilic infiltration 48 h after challenge between W/W^v and +/+ mice has been confirmed by 3 different experiments (data not shown). Our present finding is in contrast with the previous studies by Brusselle et al. [11] and Takeda et al. [12]. They found no difference in lung eosinophilia between +/+ and W/W^v mice. The discrepancy may result from the different experimental protocols. Mice were challenged with inhalated OVA for 7 and 3 constitutive days in the studies made by Brusselle et al. [11] and Takeda et al. [12]. Instead, mice were challenged only once in our study, in which detection of the contribution of mast cells in airway eosinophilia may become easier. The detection of airway obstruction in our model warrants further examination and is currently underway.

To further analyze the contribution of CD4+ T cells and mast cells to airway eosinophilia, the effects of GK1.5 and TRFK-5 were next examined. A representative result is shown in table 1. Administration of GK1.5 significantly decreased the number of eosinophils recovered in BALF of W/W^v mice 48 and 96 h after antigen challenge and that of +/+ mice 96 h after challenge, indicating that eosinophil accumulation in the lung after antigen challenge was solely dependent on CD4+ T cells. In contrast, eosinophil infiltration in +/+ mice 48 h after antigen chal-

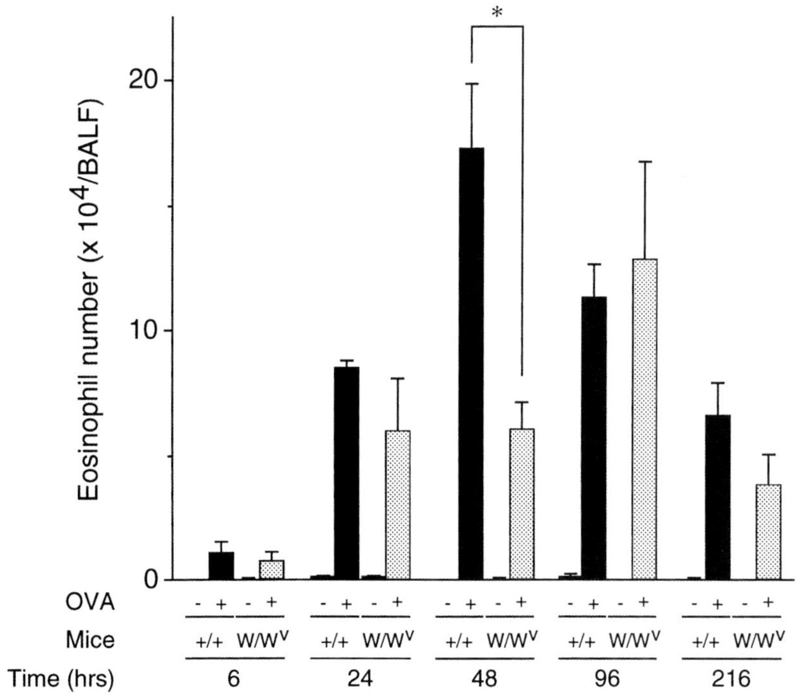

Fig. 1. Kinetics of antigen-induced eosinophil infiltration in W/W^v and +/+ mice. OVA-sensitized mice were challenged with inhaled antigen or saline for 20 min. Eosinophil number recovered in BALF 6 to 216 h after challenge: □ = saline-challenged +/+ mice; ■ = OVA-challenged +/+ mice; ▨ = saline-challenged W/W^v mice; ▩ = OVA-challenged W/W^v mice. * $p < 0.05$, compared with OVA-challenged +/+ mice.

lenge was suppressed by only ~ 50% by CD4+ T cell ablation, suggesting that mast cells significantly but only slightly contributed to eosinophilic infiltration during the limited time period of the response.

Among T cell cytokines, IL-5 has recently been reported to play an essential role in eosinophilic inflammation [3, 4, 7]. Nevertheless, many investigators have reported that mast cells secrete cytokines, including IL-5, in vitro [8, 9]. Therefore, we next examined the effect of TRFK-5 on antigen-induced eosinophil accumulation in W/W^v and +/+ mice. Airway eosinophilia in W/W^v mice 48 and 96 h after provocation was almost completely suppressed by TRFK-5, while the inhibitory effect of administration of the same antibody to +/+ mice was partial 48 h after antigen challenge, and the effect was almost the same as that of GK1.5. The crucial role of IL-5 in airway eosinophilia and hyperresponsiveness induced by antigen challenge has been clearly demonstrated by IL-5-deficient mice [13], while other factors may be generated locally and also facilitate the development of widespread eosinophilic inflammation. Mast cells can produce eosinophil-active chemical mediators, chemokines and cytokines other than IL-5 [8, 10]. Levi-Schaffer et al. [10] reported

Table 1. Effects of anti-CD4 and anti-IL-5 antibodies on antigen-induced eosinophil infiltration in W/W^v and +/+ mice

Mice	Treatment	Eosinophil number, × 10^4/BALF	
		48 h	96 h
+/+	Saline	0.2±0.1**	0.0±0.0**
+/+	OVA	17.2±0.7	12.9±1.8
+/+	OVA + GK1.5	6.9±2.9**	2.1±0.4**
+/+	OVA + TRFK-5	8.0±1.8**	1.7±1.2**
W/W^v	Saline	0.3±0.2##	0.1±0.1##
W/W^v	OVA	9.1±0.9	12.3±2.4
W/W^v	OVA + GK1.5	1.7±0.5##	1.5±0.5##
W/W^v	OVA + TRFK-5	1.5±0.4##	0.8±0.4##

OVA-sensitized mice were challenged with inhaled antigen or saline for 20 min. Either anti-murine CD4 monoclonal antibody (GK1.5, 1 mg) or anti-murine IL-5 monoclonal antibody (TRFK-5, 100 μg) was injected intravenously 6 days or 5 min before antigen challenge. Eosinophil number in BALF 48 or 96 h after challenge is shown (N = 4–8). ** $p < 0.01$ compared with OVA-challenged control +/+ mice; ## $p < 0.01$ compared with OVA-challenged control W/W^v mice.

that TNF-α produced by mast cells enhances human eosinophil survival in vitro. Renzetti et al. [14] found that a potent antagonist of TNF-α, Ro452081, markedly reduced the antigen-induced eosinophil infiltration in guinea pigs and rats 24 h after antigen challenge. These reports suggest that TNF-α may be a mediator of allergic inflammation at the early stage after antigen challenge. In addition, peptide leukotriene antagonists, MK-571 and ONO-1078, were reported to inhibit antigen-induced eosinophil accumulation in guinea pigs 8 and 24 h after antigen challenge, respectively [15, 16], suggesting that peptide leukotrienes produced by mast cells may also participate in early eosinophilic infiltration. Studies of these agents in our murine model will clarify the mechanisms of eosinophil recruitment by the mast-cell-dependent pathway, and are currently under way.

In conclusion, CD4+ T cells are functionally essential in the development of antigen-induced airway eosinophilic inflammation which is mediated by IL-5. Mast cells are also involved in airway eosinophilia, although their contribution appears partial and transient. Studies directed toward the regulation of CD4+ T cell- and IL-5-dependent eosinophilic inflammation may facilitate the development of therapeutic agents for allergic disorders including asthma and atopic dermatitis.

References

1 Corrigan CJ, Kay AB: T cells and eosinophils in the pathogenesis of asthma. Immunol Today 1992;13:501–507.
2 Kay AB, 'Helper' (CD4+) T cells and eosinophils in allergy and asthma. Am Rev Respir Dis 1992;145:S22–S26.
3 Mori A, Suko M, Nishizaki Y, Kaminuma O, Kobayashi S, Matsuzaki G, Yamamoto K, Ito K, Tsuruoka N, Okudaira H: IL-5 production by CD4+ T cells of asthmatic patients is suppressed by glucocorticoids and immunosuppressants FK506 and cyclosporin A. Int Immunol 1995;7:449–457.
4 Mori A, Kaminuma O, Suko M, Mikami T, Nishizaki Y, Ohmura T, Hoshino A, Asakura Y, Miyazawa K, Ando T, Okumura Y, Yamamoto K, Okudaira H: Cellular and molecular mechanisms of IL-5 synthesis in atopic diseases: A study with allergen-specific human helper T cells. J Allergy Clin Immunol 1997; 100:S56–64.
5 Nakajima H, Iwamoto I, Tomoe S, Matsumura R, Tomioka H, Takatsu K, Yoshida S: CD4+ T-lymphocytes and interleukin-5 mediate antigen-induced eosinophil infiltration into the mouse trachea. Am Rev Respir Dis 1992;146: 374–377.
6 Gavett SH, Chen X, Finkelman F, Wills-Karp M: Depletion of murine CD4+ T lymphocytes prevents antigen-induced airway hyperreactivity and pulmonary eosinophilia. Am J Respir Cell Mol Biol 1994;10:587–593.
7 Kaminuma O, Mori A, Ogawa K, Nakata A, Kikkawa H, Naito K, Suko M, Okudaira H: Successful transfer of late phase eosinophil infiltration in the lung by infusion of helper T cell clones. Am J Respir Cell Mol Biol 1997;16: 448–454.
8 Plaut M, Pierce JH, Watson CJ, Hanley-Hyde J, Nordan RP, Paul WE: Mast cell lines produce lymphokines in response to cross-linkage of Fcε RI or to calcium ionophores. Nature 1989;339:64–67.
9 Okayama Y, Petit-Frere C, Kassel O, Semper A, Quint D, Tunon-de-Lara MJ, Bradding P, Holgate ST, Church MK: IgE-dependent expression of mRNA for IL-4 and IL-5 in human lung mast cells. J Immunol 1995;155:1796–1808.
10 Levi-Schaffer F, Temkin V, Malamud V, Feld S, Zilberman Y: Mast cells enhance eosinophil survival in vitro: Role of TNF-α and granulocyte-macrophage colony-stimulating factor. J Immunol 1998;160:5554–5562.
11 Brusselle GG, Kips JC, Tavernier JH, van der Heyden JG, Cuvelier CA, Pauwels RA, Bluethmann H: Attenuation of allergic airway inflammation in IL-4 deficient mice. Clin Exp Allergy 1994;24:73–80.
12 Takeda K, Hamelmann E, Joetham A, Shultz LD, Larsen GL, Irvin CG, Gelfand EW: Development of eosinophilic airway inflammation and airway hyperresponsiveness in mast cell-deficient mice. J Exp Med 1997;186:449–454.
13 Foster PS, Hogan SP, Ramsay AJ, Matthaei KI, Young IG: Interleukin-5 deficiency abolishes eosinophilia, airways hyperreactivity, and lung damage in a mouse asthma model. J Exp Med 1996;183:195–201.
14 Renzetti LM, Paciorek PM, Tannu SA, Rinaldi NC, Tocker JE, Wasserman MA, Gater PR: Pharmacological evidence for tumor necrosis factor as a mediator of allergic inflammation in the airway. J Pharmacol Exp Ther 1996;278: 847–853.
15 Foster A, Chan CC: Peptide leukotriene involvement in pulmonary eosinophil migration upon antigen challenge in the actively sensitized guinea pig. Int Arch Allergy Appl Immunol 1991;96:279–284.
16 Itoh K, Takahashi E, Mukaiyama O, Satoh Y, Yamaguchi T: Effects of thromboxane synthase inhibitor (CS-518) on the eosinophil-dependent late asthmatic response and airway hyperresponsiveness in guinea pigs. Int Arch Allergy Immunol 1996;109:79–85.

International Archives of
Allergy and
Immunology

Int Arch Allergy Immunol 1999;120(suppl 1):19–23

IL-4 Induces Eotaxin in Human Dermal Fibroblasts

Mitsuru Mochizuki[a,b] Jens-M. Schröder[b] Enno Christophers[b]
Shoso Yamamoto[a]

[a]Department of Dermatology, Hiroshima University School of Medicine, Hiroshima, Japan;
[b]Department of Dermatology, University of Kiel, Germany

Key Words
Eotaxin · Eosinophil · Chemokine · IL-4 · Fibroblast

Abstract
A common feature of Th2-mediated skin diseases is selective eosinophil (Eo) infiltration in the affected dermis. However, the mechanisms of selective Eo recruitment are not yet fully understood. Our recent findings indicated that dermal fibroblasts actively participate in the accumulation of Eo in Th2-mediated skin inflammation. Following stimulation with IL-4, dermal fibroblasts produce eotaxin, which is the only biologically active Eo attractant detected in the supernatants. Natural eotaxin is comprised of a mixture of N-terminal-truncated and *O*-glycosylated variants. The expression of eotaxin mRNA is upregulated within 1 h after stimulation. TNF-α markedly enhances eotaxin mRNA expression and release of the protein product from IL-4-stimulated fibroblasts. As mast cells and Th2 cells produce both cytokines, it is probable that Eo recruitment into sites of allergen-induced, Th2-mediated skin reactions is, at least in part, due to IL-4-stimulated induction of eotaxin in dermal fibroblasts.

Selective eosinophil (Eo) infiltration is a common feature of allergic diseases such as bronchial asthma, allergic rhinitis, and atopic dermatitis. Eo infiltrate the dermis in allergen-induced late-phase skin reaction in atopic subjects [1]. In the lesional skin of patients with atopic dermatitis, dermal deposition of Eo major basic protein was demonstrated [2].

The mechanisms of selective Eo recruitment are not yet fully understood. Clinical and experimental observations have suggested an association between tissue eosinophilia and Th2 cytokines. Together with Eo, the Th2 cytokines IL-4 and IL-5 have been detected in bronchoalveolar lavage fluid or bronchial biopsy specimens from patients with bronchial asthma [3], and in the sites of allergen-induced late-phase skin reactions [4]. IL-4 and IL-5 play critical roles in mobilizing Eo to these sites, but the presence of these cytokines alone is insufficient to induce accumulation of Eo in the tissue. In addition, supernatants of blood- and tissue-derived Th2 clones showed no significant Eo chemotactic activity in the Boyden chamber chemotaxis assay system [unpubl. obs.]. These observations suggest that cells other than Th2 lymphocytes produce a factor(s) which directly attracts Eo in Th2-mediated conditions.

Chemokines comprise a family of small proteins that have been implicated in the selective recruitment of leukocyte subsets. Eotaxin is the only chemokine described

KARGER

Fax + 41 61 306 12 34
E-Mail karger@karger.ch
www.karger.com

1018–2438/99/1205–0019$17.50/0

Accessible online at:
http://BioMedNet.com/karger

Mitsuru Mochizuki, MD
Department of Dermatology, Hiroshima University School of Medicine
Kasumi 1-2-3, Minami-ku, Hiroshima 734-8551 (Japan)
Tel. +81 82 257 5238, Fax +81 82 257 5239
E-Mail mitzuru@ipc.hiroshima-u.ac.jp

	1 · · · 5 · · · 10 · · · 15 · · · 20 · · · 25 · · · 30 · · · 35 · ·
human Eotaxin	GPASVPTTCCFNLANRKIPLQRLESYRRITSGKCPQK
natural Eotaxin	GPASVPTTCCFNLANRKIPLQRLESYRRITSGKCPQK
	40% (G) 50% (A) 10% (S)
	· · 40 · · · 45 · · · 50 · · · 55 · · · 60 · · · 65 · · · 70 · · ·
human Eotaxin	AVIFKTKLAKDICADPKKKWVQDSMKYLDQKSPTPKP
natural Eotaxin	AVIFKTKLAKDICADPKKKWVQDSMKYLDQKSPXPKP

Fig. 1. Complete amino acid sequence analysis of natural eotaxin β. the deduced sequence of human eotaxin is aligned for comparison. Percentages at residues 1, 3, and 4 indicate the amount of N-terminal variants starting with the respective residue. Residue 71 was not determined by Edman degradation, and *O*-glycosylation at this residue is speculated.

to date that acts on a single receptor, CCR3, which is present in high numbers on Eo [5]. Thus, human eotaxin represents an attractive candidate cytokine to explain the selective accumulation of Eo in tissue. However, whether eotaxin is actually produced in Th2-mediated conditions is not clear. Recently, we found that biologically active eotaxin is produced by dermal fibroblasts stimulated with IL-4, which suggests the involvement of eotaxin in skin diseases [6]. Here we briefly summarize our observations and discuss the role of eotaxin in Eo infiltration into the lesional skin of Th2-mediated inflammation.

Dermal Fibroblasts as a Source of Eo Attractants

As the dermis is the main focus of tissue eosinophilia in cutaneous allergic inflammation, dermal rather than epidermal cells may contribute to Eo infiltration in skin inflammation. Previous studies indicated that dermal fibroblasts, the major cellular component of dermis, express the mRNAs encoding the Eo-specific chemokines RANTES [7], eotaxin [8], MCP-3 [unpubl. data], and MCP-4 [9], and that bioactive RANTES is produced by TNF-α-stimulated dermal fibroblasts [10]. Recently, we found that dermal fibroblasts secrete bioactive eotaxin and RANTES 3 days after stimulation with TNF-α [11]. However, the effect of Th2-mediated conditions on the production of these chemokines remains to be investigated.

IL-4 Induces the Release of Eotaxin from Dermal Fibroblasts

Supernatants of foreskin-derived fibroblasts contained Eo-chemotactic activity when cultured in the presence of 20 ng/ml of IL-4 for 48 h. Biochemical characterization revealed that the Eo attractants completely bound to a heparin-Sepharose column, and that the nonbinding proteins and lipids in the effluent showed no significant Eo chemotactic activity. Further purification of the heparin-binding Eo chemotactic proteins by reversed-phase HPLC resulted in a single peak, which migrated as a single band on SDS-PAGE with an apparent molecular mass of 13 kD. Amino acid sequence analysis revealed the presence of three N-termini starting with Ala-Ser-Val (50%), Gly-Pro-Ala-Ser-Val (40%) and Ser-Val (10%) (fig. 1). The complete amino acid sequence of the purified material was determined by N-terminal sequencing of peptide fragments which were obtained from the material after digestion with various endoproteinases. This protein was shown to be identical to the predicted sequence of human eotaxin. Consistent with natural eotaxin purified from TNF-α-stimulated dermal fibroblasts, *O*-glycosylation at threonine residue 71 was indicated by glycan ELISA and mass spectrometry of peptide mapping fragments (fig. 1). Purified eotaxin showed a specific chemotactic activity for Eo similar to recombinant and TNF-α-stimulated fibroblast-derived eotaxin.

By semiquantitative reverse transcriptase PCR, we found that IL-4 enhanced eotaxin mRNA expression in dermal fibroblasts in a dose- and time-dependent manner. Half-maximum expression occurred after stimulation with 0.1 ng/ml of IL-4. The expression was upregulated within 1 h and showed maximum response after 18 h.

While both eotaxin and RANTES are released from TNF-α-stimulated fibroblasts, eotaxin is the only Eo attractant released from IL-4-stimulated dermal fibroblasts (fig. 2a). The other known Eo attractants RANTES and MCP-4 were not detected as either bioactive or immunoreactive proteins. MCP-3 mRNA expression was strong, but no release of the protein was detected in the supernatants. It is noteworthy that the expression of chemokine mRNA did not necessarily indicate the release of natural bioactive products.

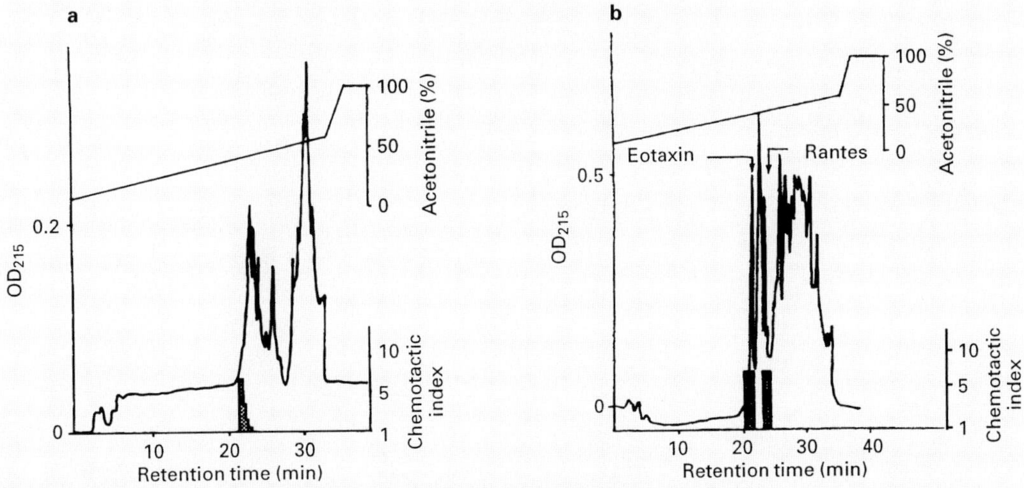

Fig. 2. Fibroblasts release a single Eo attractant upon IL-4 stimulation (**a**). A combination of IL-4 and TNF-α strongly stimulates the release of eotaxin and also stimulates the production of RANTES (**b**). Preparative RP-HPLC of heparin-bound proteins secreted by stimulated fibroblasts is shown. The amount of the starting materials was equal for both preparations.

TNF-α in Combination with IL-4 Strongly Increases the Release of Different Eotaxin Variants

On stimulation of fibroblasts with IL-4 (20 ng/ml) together with TNF-α (20 ng/ml), the expression of eotaxin mRNA was highly upregulated, and 10- to 20-fold greater amounts of eotaxin were released into the supernatant. Under these conditions, bioactive RANTES was also produced (fig. 2b). Three biochemically different eotaxin isoforms, termed eotaxins α, β, and γ, were separated by micro-Mono S-HPLC and micro-RP-HPLC (fig. 3). Of these, eotaxin α accounted for 60% of total eotaxin. Chemotaxis assay revealed that eotaxin α was the most potent, and that isoforms β and γ were slightly less potent. However, maximum Eo migration induced by each isoform was similar. Each fraction of eotaxin isoforms contained three N-terminal variants as seen in IL-4-stimulated fibroblast-derived eotaxin, and all isoforms were shown to be glycosylated. The comparison of peptide mapping patterns seen after digestion of each isoform with endopeptidase Lys C indicated that eotaxin derived from IL-4-stimulated fibroblasts was identical to eotaxin β. We speculated that the different purified variants were the result of differences in glycosylation and derivatization.

A Possible Mechanism of Eosinophil Recruitment in Th2-Mediated Skin Diseases

Originally, RANTES appeared to be significantly involved as an attractant in Eo tissue accumulation. Indeed, dermal fibroblasts produce high levels of biologically active RANTES after stimulation with TNF-α [10]. However, in allergic lung inflammation in mice, eosinophilic infiltration appeared to be dependent on the presence of T cells, but not RANTES [12]. In addition, RANTES mRNA expression shows no correlation with Eo tissue infiltration in allergen-induced cutaneous late-phase responses [13]. Th1-type cytokines are also known to induce RANTES secretion from epithelial cells, and Th2 cytokines inhibit the production of RANTES [14]. Eotaxin was first purified from the bronchoalveolar lavage fluid of sensitized guinea pigs after allergen challenge [15] and is the only eosinophil-specific chemokine shown to bind exclusively to the CCR3 chemokine receptor to date. Although the expression of eotaxin mRNA and its immunoreactivity were reported in human tissues, it had remained unclear whether bioactive eotaxin actually plays a role in Eo infiltration in tissues [16]. In mice, there is a remarkable Eo infiltration when IL-4-producing tumor cells are transplanted into the skin [17], and eotaxin mRNA is upregulated at the site [18]. Our results indicate

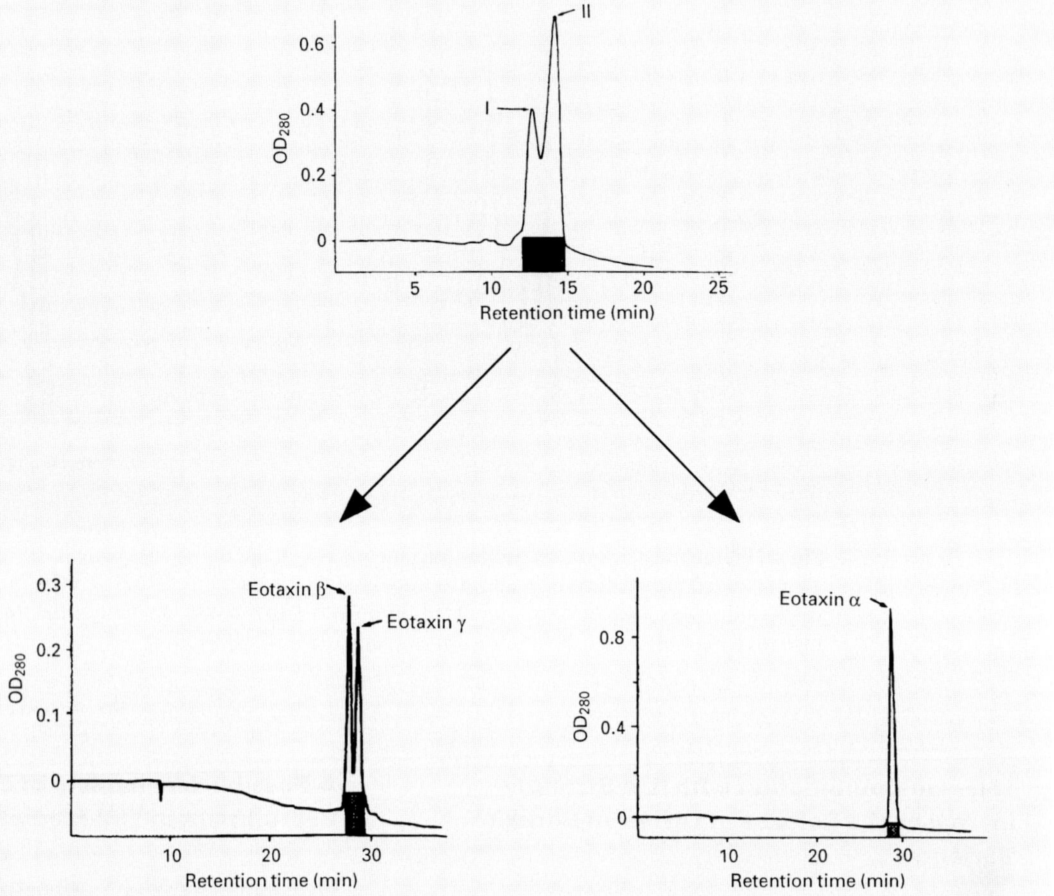

Fig. 3. Eotaxin variants released from fibroblasts stimulated by IL-4 and TNF-α. Micro-Mono S-HPLC of the eotaxin-containing fraction (fig. 2b peak 'eotaxin') resulted in two protein peaks (peak I and II). They were further separated upon micro-RP 18-HPLC. Peak I resulted in two bioactive protein peaks (eotaxin β and γ), and peak II led to one bioactive protein peak (eotaxin α).

that eotaxin is the only bioactive Eo attractant produced by IL-4-stimulated human fibroblasts. Recent in vivo observations also emphasized the role of eotaxin in Th2-mediated skin inflammation. Intradermal injection of IL-4 in rats induced eotaxin mRNA expression at the site of injection, beginning at 4 h and reaching a maximum at 18 h. Anti-eotaxin antibodies inhibited the late-phase (24–48 h) but not the early-phase (0–4 h) Eo accumulation after IL-4 injection [19], suggesting the involvement of eotaxin in the late-phase reaction.

The observation that a combination of IL-4 and TNF-α induces the release of large amounts of eotaxin is of particular importance because mast cells release both of these cytokines on IgE-dependent stimulation [20]. In cutaneous allergic reactions, immediate reactions are often followed by Eo several hours later. As eotaxin mRNA is upregulated within 1 h after IL-4 stimulation, fibroblast-derived eotaxin may play a critical role in Eo accumulation in these conditions. This cytokine combination is also known to strongly enhance the expression of VCAM-1 on vascular endothelial cells [21]. It is thus possible that the Eo infiltration observed in allergen-induced late-phase skin reactions is induced by mast cell-derived IL-4 and TNF-α in concert with eotaxin from fibroblasts stimulated with these cytokines.

Our findings explain, at least in part, the selective recruitment of Eo into affected skin in Th2-mediated skin inflammation.

References

1 Gaga M, Frew AJ, Varney VA, Kay AB: Eosinophil activation and T lymphocyte infiltration in allergen-induced late phase skin reactions and classical delayed-type hypersensitivity. J Immunol 1991;147:816–822.

2 Leiferman KM: A current perspective on the role of eosinophils in dermatologic diseases. J Am Acad Dermatol 1991;24:1101–1112.

3 Robinson DS, Hamid Q, Ying S, Tsicopoulos A, Barkans J, Bentley AM, Corrigan C, Durham SR, Kay AB: Predominant TH2-like bronchoalveolar T-lymphocyte population in atopic asthma. N Engl J Med 1992;326:298–304.

4 Vowels BR, Rook AH, Cassin M, Zweiman B: Expression of interleukin-4 and interleukin-5 mRNA in developing cutaneous late-phase reactions. J Allergy Clin Immunol 1995;96:92–96.

5 Heath H, Qin S, Rao P, Wu L, LaRosa G, Kassam N, Ponath PD, Mackay CR: Chemokine receptor usage by human eosinophils. J Clin Invest 1997;99:178–184.

6 Mochizuki M, Bartels J, Mallet AI, Christophers E, Schröder JM: IL-4 induces eotaxin: A possible mechanism of selective eosinophil recruitment in helminth infection and atopy. J Immunol 1998;160:60–68.

7 Sticherling M, Kupper M, Koltrowiz F, Bronscheuer E, Kulke R, Klinger M, Kameyoshi Y, Christophers E, Schröder M: Detection of the chemokine RANTES in cytokine-stimulated human dermal fibroblasts. J Invest Dermatol 1995;105:585–591.

8 Bartels J, Sculter C, Richter E, Noso N, Kulke R, Christophers E, Schröder M: Human dermal fibroblasts express eotaxin: Molecular cloning, mRNA expression, and identification of eotaxin sequence variants. Biochem Biophys Commun 1996;225:1045–1051.

9 Petering H, Hochstetter R, Kimming D, Smolarski R, Kapp A, Elsner J: Detection of MCP-4 in dermal fibroblasts and its activation of the respiratory burst in human eosinophils. J Immunol 1998;160:555–558.

10 Noso N, Sticherling M, Bartels J, Mallet AI, Christophers E, Schröder M: Identification of an N-terminally truncated form of the chemokine RANTES and granulocyte-macrophage colony-stimulating factor as major eosinophil attractants released by cytokine-stimulated dermal fibroblasts. J Immunol 1996;156:1946–1953.

11 Noso N, Bartels J, Mallet AI, Mochizuki M, Christophers E, Schröder JM: Delayed production of biologically active O-glycosylated forms of human eotaxin by tumor-necrosis-factor-α-stimulated dermal fibroblasts. Eur J Biochem 1998;253:114–122.

12 MacLean JA, Ownbey R, Luster AD: T cell-dependent regulation of eotaxin in allergen-induced pulmonary eosinophilia. J Exp Med 1996;184:1461–1469.

13 Ying S, Taborda-Barata L, Meng Q, Humbert M, Kay AB: The kinetics of allergen-induced transcription of messenger RNA for monocyte chemotactic protein-3 and RANTES in the skin of human atopic subjects: Relationship to eosinophil, T cell, and macrophage recruitment. J Exp Med 1995;181:2153–2159.

14 Marfaing-Koka A, Devergne O, Gorgone G, Portier A, Schall TJ, Galanaud P, Emilie D: Regulation of the production of the RANTES chemokine by endothelial cells. J Immunol 1995;154:1870–1878.

15 Griffiths-Johnson DA, Collins PD, Rossi AG, Jose PJ, Williams TJ: The chemokine eotaxin activates guinea-pig eosinophils in vitro and causes their accumulation into the lung in vivo. Biochem Biophys Commun 1993;197:1167–1172.

16 Ponath PD, Qin S, Ringer DJ, Clark-Lewis I, Wang J, Kassam N, Smith H, Shi X, Gonzalo JA, Newman W, Gutierrez-Ramos JC, Mackay CR: Cloning of the human eosinophil chemoattractant, eotaxin. J Clin Invest 1996;97:604–612.

17 Tepper RI, Pattengale PK, Leder P: Murine interleukin-4 displays potent anti-tumor activity in vivo. Cell 1989;57:503–512.

18 Rothenberg ME, Luster AD, Leder P: Murine eotaxin: An eosinophil chemoattractant inducible in endothelial cells and in interleukin 4-induced tumor suppression. Proc Natl Acad Sci USA 1995;92:8960–8964.

19 Sanz MJ, Ponath PD, Mackay CR, Newman W, Miyasaka M, Tamatani T, Flanagan BF, Lobb RR, Williams TJ, Nourshargh S, Jose PJ: Human eotaxin induces α4 and β2 integrin-dependent eosinophil accumulation in rat skin in vivo: Delayed generation of eotaxin in response to IL-4. J Immunol 1998;160:3569–3576.

20 Steffen M, Abboud M, Potter GK, Yung XP, Moore MAS: Presence of tumor necrosis factor on a related factor in human basophil/mast cells. Immunology 1989;66:445–450.

21 Barks JL, McQuillan JJ, Iademarco MF: TNF-α and IL-4 synergically increase vascular cell adhesion molecule-1 expression in cultured vascular smooth muscle cells. J Immunol 1997;159:4532–4538.

International Archives of
Allergy and
Immunology

Int Arch Allergy Immunol 1999;120(suppl 1):24–26

Regulatory Mechanisms of Eosinophil Adhesion to and Transmigration across Endothelial Cells by α_4 and β_2 Integrins

Hideaki Yamamoto Makoto Nagata

Pulmonary Division, Second Department of Internal Medicine, Saitama Medical School, Irumagun, Saitama, Japan

Key Words
Eosinophil · Endothelial cells · Cell adhesion · Transendothelial migration · Adhesion molecules

Abstract
To participate in allergic airway inflammation, it is necessary for blood eosinophils (Eos) to adhere to and migrate across pulmonary vascular endothelial cells (EC). Accumulating evidence has established that Eos adhesion molecules, such as α_4 and β_2 integrins, play central roles in these processes. We have reported that Eos spontaneously adhere to recombinant human (rh)-VCAM-1, while adhesion to rh-ICAM-1 requires a second stimulus such as GM-CSF. Furthermore, our study employing human pulmonary microvascular endothelial cells (HPMEC) revealed that although the α_4 integrin/VCAM-1 pathway is crucial for the firm adhesion of Eos, subsequent transendothelial migration occurred dependent on the β_2 integrin/ICAM-1 pathway. We also discuss secretagogues that would affect Eos recruitment to the airways via regulation of α_4 and β_2 integrins.

Eosinophils (Eos) are pivotal effector cells in the development of airway inflammation in bronchial asthma. The mechanisms by which Eos preferentially accumulate to the asthmatic airways are not completely established. To recruit into the asthmatic airways, it is necessary for peripheral blood Eos to adhere to and then migrate across pulmonary vascular endothelial cells (EC). It is generally accepted that these two processes are mediated by Eos integrin adhesion molecules including α_4 integrins such as $\alpha_4\beta_1$ (CD49d/CD29; VLA-4) and $\alpha_4\beta_7$, and β_2 integrins such as $\alpha_L\beta_2$ (CD11a/CD18; LFA-1) and $\alpha_M\beta_2$ (CD11b/CD18; Mac-1) [1]. The counterligands expressed on EC for α_4 and β_2 integrins are VCAM-1 and ICAM-1, respectively. Since all leukocytes can utilize the β_2 integrin/ICAM-1 pathway for their adhesion and transendothelial migration, it is proposed that the α_4 integrin, expressed on Eos but not on neutrophils, plays a key role in the development of selective Eos recruitment to the airways [2]. For example, in the case of Eos, but not in that of neutrophils, adhesion to IL-1-stimulated EC is blocked by anti-α_4 integrin or anti-VCAM-1 mAb in vitro [3, 4]. However, the contribution of the α_4 integrin/VCAM-1 pathway to the subsequent Eos transendothelial migration remains to be defined [5–7].

Current understanding regarding Eos interaction with EC is largely derived from the study of human umbilical vein endothelial cells (HUVEC), a macrovascular nonpulmonary cell [2–7]. Human pulmonary microvascular endothelial cells (HPMEC) are likely to be more relevant than HUVEC as an in vitro model of cell trafficking to the lung; this assumption is based on the observation that

KARGER

Fax + 41 61 306 12 34
E-Mail karger@karger.ch
www.karger.com

1018–2438/99/1205–0024$17.50/0

Accessible online at:
http://BioMedNet.com/karger

Makoto Nagata, MD
Pulmonary Division, Second Department of Internal Medicine
Saitama Medical School, 38 Morohongo, Moroyamacho
Irumagun, Saitama 350-0495 (Japan)
Tel. +81 492 76 1319, Fax +81 492 95 8399, E-Mail favre4mn@saitama-med.ac.jp

Table 1. Effect of cytokine(s) on adhesion molecule expression on HPMEC and the influence of these molecules on Eos adhesion and transmigration

	Medium	IL-1β	TNF-α	TNF-α + IL-4
HPMEC expression of				
ICAM-1[a]	+	+++	+++	+++
VCAM-1[a]	–	+	++	+++
Adhesion[b]	+/–	+	++	+++ α_4 integrin
Transmigration[b]	+/–	+++ β_2 integrin	++	+

[a] HPMEC monolayers were treated with medium, IL-1β (6 h), TNF-α (24 h), or TNF-α + IL-4 (24 h) (all at 100 p*M*), and ICAM-1 and VCAM-1 expression was determined.
[b] Eos adhesion to and transmigration across medium or cytokine(s)-pretreated HPMEC monolayers were determined.
+++ = very strong; ++ = strong; + = moderate; – = not detected.

macro- and microvascular EC have considerable heterogeneity in their biological properties [8]. We have examined the involvement of α_4 and β_2 integrins in Eos adhesion and transendothelial migration with HPMEC monolayers (table 1) [9]. HPMEC expressed ICAM-1 (8% positive cells by flow cytometry), but not VCAM-1, constitutively. More than 80% of HPMEC expressed ICAM-1 when they were stimulated with IL-1β or TNF-α (+/– IL-4). VCAM-1 expression, however, varied with cytokine treatment, and the order of potency was as follows: TNF-α + IL-4 > TNF-α > IL-1β. Eos adhesion to these cytokine-treated HPMEC followed the same order as that observed for VCAM-1 expression: TNF-α + IL-4 > TNF-α > IL-1β. Interestingly, Eos transmigration across the HPMEC monolayer occurred inversely with regard to VCAM-1 expression on, and Eos adhesion to, HPMEC: IL-1β > TNF-α > TNF-α + IL-4. The highest adhesion (TNF-α + IL-4-stimulated HPMEC) was inhibited by anti-α_4 integrin mAb, while anti-β_2 integrin mAb alone had no effect. In agreement with previous studies employing HUVEC, transendothelial migration was inhibited by anti-β_2 integrin mAb [5–7]. These results suggest that α_4 integrin/VCAM interaction is important for Eos adhesion, and that subsequent transmigration is dependent on β_2 integrin/ICAM-1. Kuijpers et al. [10] reported that 'freezing' β_1 integrin in a state of high avidity by activating mAb completely inhibited Eos migration across endothelial-cell-coated filters. Therefore, it is possible that although the α_4 integrin/VCAM-1 pathway is crucial for Eos adhesion, the firm adhesion via this pathway may, in such static experimental conditions, attenuate subsequent transmigration. It has also been reported that in vivo blocking of the α_4 integrin/VCAM-1 pathway prevents antigen-induced Eos infiltration into the lung in an animal model of asthma [11]. Thus, in a blood-flowing condition, inhibition of the α_4 integrin/VCAM-1 pathway may be sufficient to attenuate Eos trafficking to the lung.

To investigate the factor(s) responsible for inducing Eos transendothelial migration following adhesion via α_4 integrin/VCAM-1 is of great interest. Weber et al. [12] reported the differential regulation of β_1 and β_2 integrin avidity of Eos by RANTES and MCP-3. These C-C chemokines rapidly increased and then subsequently reduced Eos adhesiveness of α_4 integrin for VCAM-1. These effects were dependent on actin polymerization, and the deactivation of α_4 integrin leads to cell detachment. In contrast, C-C chemokines stimulated a prolonged increase in the adhesiveness of β_2 integrin for ICAM-1 through a conformational change of this integrin. Thus, the regulation of a transient α_4 integrin/VCAM-1-dependent Eos adhesion to, and a rapid detachment from, HPMEC by C-C chemokines may allow Eos to undergo β_2 integrin/ICAM-1-dependent transmigration successfully.

Regulation of Eos β_2 integrin may be triggered by α_4-integrin-dependent adhesion of Eos with VCAM-1. It has been suggested that Eos adhesion to VCAM-1 is an important step not only for selective accumulation of Eos but also for determining eventual effector functions of airway Eos. We have previously observed that Eos spontaneously adhere to recombinant human (rh)-VCAM-1, while Eos adhesion to rh-ICAM-1 requires a second stimulus such as GM-CSF or platelet-activating factor [13]. Adhesion to rh-VCAM-1 resulted in the generation of superoxide anion from Eos [14]. Superoxide anion generation from

Eos in response to VCAM-1 was significantly inhibited by anti-α_4 integrin mAb. Interestingly, anti-β_2 integrin also inhibited VCAM-1-induced superoxide anion generation without affecting cell adhesion, suggesting that the signaling via the α_4 integrin/VCAM-1 pathway resulted in modulation of β_2 integrin. Moreover, we recently observed that H_2O_2, one of the reactive oxygen species, induces Eos adhesion to EC via increased expression of β_2 integrins [15], raising the possibility that the process of respiratory burst may further augment the upregulation of Eos β_2 integrins in an autocrine and/or paracrine fashion. These observations suggest that Eos adhesion to EC as well as subsequent activation via α_4 integrin/VCAM-1 may upregulate β_2 integrins. This Eos with upregulated β_2 integrin may migrate across EC efficiently and then degranulate in the airways [16].

Eos adhesion to and transmigration across EC comprise an initial step of Eos recruitment to the inflammation site, and these processes are achieved by a complex of several factors, including adhesion molecules, inflammatory mediators, chemoattractants and cytokines [17]. Eos α_4 and β_2 integrins are most likely the essential adhesion molecules involved in these processes. Further investigations are required to establish the exact regulatory mechanisms of α_4 and β_2 integrins of Eos in allergic inflammation.

References

1 Carlos TM, Harlan JM: Leukocyte-endothelial adhesion molecules. Blood 1994;84:2068–2101.

2 Weller PF, Rand TH, Goelz SE, Chi-Rosso G, Lobb RR: Human eosinophil adherence to vascular endothelium mediated by binding to vascular cell adhesion molecule 1 and endothelial leukocyte adhesion molecule 1. Proc Natl Acad Sci USA 1991;88:7430–7433.

3 Walsh GM, Mermod J-J, Hartnell A, Kay AB, Wardlaw AJ: Human eosinophil, but not neutrophil, adherence to IL-1-stimulated human umbilical vascular endothelial cells is $\alpha_4\beta_1$ (very late antigen-4) dependent. J Immunol 1991;146:3419–3423.

4 Bochner BS, Luscinskas FW, Gimbrone MA, Newman W, Sterbinsky SA, Derse-Anthony CP, Klunk D, Schleimer RP: Adhesion of human basophils, eosinophils, and neutrophils to interleukin 1-activated human vascular endothelial cells: Contributions of endothelial cell adhesion molecules. J Exp Med 1991;173:1553–1556.

5 Moser R, Fehr J, Olgiati L, Bruijnzeel PLB: Migration of primed human eosinophils across cytokine-activated endothelial cell monolayers. Blood 1992;79:2937–2945.

6 Moser R, Fehr J, Bruijnzeel PLB: IL-4 controls the selective endothelium-driven transmigration of eosinophils from allergic individuals. J Immunol 1992;149:1432–1438.

7 Ebisawa M, Bochner BS, Georas SN, Schleimer RP: Eosinophil transendothelial migration induced by cytokines. I. Role of endothelial and eosinophil adhesion molecules in IL-1β-induced transendothelial migration. J Immunol 1992;149:4021–4028.

8 Carley WW, Niedbala MJ, Gerritsen ME: Isolation, cultivation, and partial characterization of microvascular endothelium derived from human lung. Am J Respir Cell Mol Biol 1992;7:620–630.

9 Yamamoto H, Sedgwick JB, Busse WW: Differential regulation of eosinophil adhesion and transmigration by pulmonary microvascular endothelial cells. J Immunol 1998;161:971–977.

10 Kuijpers TW, Mul EPJ, Blom M, Kovach NL, Gaeta FCA, Tollefson V, Elices MJ, Harlan JM: Freezing adhesion molecules in a state of high-avidity binding blocks eosinophil migration. J Exp Med 1993;178:279–284.

11 Nakajima H, Sano H, Nishimura T, Yoshida S, Iwamoto I: Role of vascular cell adhesion molecule 1/very late activation antigen 4 and intercellular adhesion molecule 1/lymphocyte function-associated antigen 1 interactions in antigen-induced eosinophil and T cell recruitment into the tissue. J Exp Med 1994;179:1145–1154.

12 Weber C, Kitayama J, Springer TA: Differential regulation of β_1 and β_2 integrin avidity by chemoattractants in eosinophils. Proc Natl Acad Sci USA 1996;93:10939–10944.

13 Nagata M, Sedgwick JB, Kita H, Busse WW: Granulocyte-macrophage colony-stimulating factor augments ICAM-1 and VCAM-1 activation of eosinophil function. Am J Respir Cell Mol Biol 1998;19:158–166.

14 Nagata M, Sedgwick JB, Bates ME, Kita H, Busse WW: Eosinophil adhesion to vascular cell adhesion molecule-1 activates superoxide anion generation. J Immunol 1995;155:2194–2202.

15 Nagata M, Choo JH, Shibasaki M, Sakamoto Y, Matsuo H: H_2O_2 upregulates eosinophil adhesion to endothelial cells. J Allergy Clin Immunol 1998;101:S210.

16 Horie S, Kita H: CD11b/CD18 (Mac-1) is required for degranulation of human eosinophils induced by human recombinant granulocyte-macrophage colony-stimulating factor and platelet-activating factor. J Immunol 1994;152:5457–5467.

17 Resnick MB, Weller PF: Mechanisms of eosinophil recruitment. Am J Respir Cell Mol Biol 1993;8:349–355.

International Archives of
Allergy and
Immunology

Int Arch Allergy Immunol 1999;120(suppl 1):27–29

Whole-Blood Flow-Cytometric Analysis of Induction of Adhesion Molecules Expression on Eosinophils Stimulated by Phorbol-12-Myristate-13-Acetate/Ionomycin

Norihiro Saito[a] Hiroyuki Kayaba[a] Kohei Honda[a] Yoshiyuki Yamada[a]
Chang-Hao Cui[a] Yumiko Kamada[b] Tomoe Kuwasaki[b] Hajime Oyamada[b]
Junichi Chihara[a,b]

[a]Department of Clinical and Laboratory Medicine, Akita University School of Medicine and
[b]Division of Central Laboratory, Akita University Hospital, Akita, Japan

Key Words

Flow cytometry · Whole blood analysis · Eosinophils · Asthma · β_1, β_2 Integrin

Abstract

Background: Activation of eosinophils is closely associated with the pathology of allergic inflammatory disease, especially bronchial asthma. We recently investigated the activation of eosinophils by applying whole blood to a flow cytometer. We measured here β_1 and β_2 integrin on eosinophils stimulated by phorbol-12-myristate-13-acetate (PMA)/ionomycin to evaluate eosinophil activation in vitro using whole blood. ***Methods:*** Heparinized whole blood was diluted with the same volume of RPMI 1640, then cells were incubated in the presence or absence of PMA and ionomycin for 45 min at 37 °C. After hemolyzation with lysing solution, flow-cytometric findings for CR3, LFA1-α, LFA1-β and VLA-4 expression on eosinophils were examined. ***Results:*** Mean fluorescent intensity (MFI) of CR3 and LFA1-β stimulated by PMA and ionomycin was significantly higher than that of the unstimulated control. MFI of LFA1-α showed no significant difference from the unstimulated control. On the other hand, MFI of VLA-4 tended to decrease. ***Conclusions:*** Our method to distinguish eosinophils from various cell groups in whole blood is simple and time-saving, similar to conditions in vivo and may allow intensive investigation of eosinophils in clinical laboratories as well as in research laboratories. We are currently investigating the influence of different kinds of stimulations, regulation factors or agents on eosinophils using this method.

Introduction

It was recently recognized that atopic diseases such as bronchial asthma involve allergic inflammation, and in inflamed focuses, many types of cells, such as eosinophils, macrophages, lymphocytes, and platelets participate in the allergic inflammatory reactions. Eosinophils are considered to be the major inflammatory cells in bronchial asthma [1, 2], since eosinophil-specific granule proteins

KARGER

Fax + 41 61 306 12 34
E-Mail karger@karger.ch
www.karger.com

1018–2438/99/1205–0027$17.50/0

Accessible online at:
http://BioMedNet.com/karger

Dr. Junichi Chihara
Department of Clinical and Laboratory Medicine
1-1-1 Hondo
Akita 010 (Japan)
Tel. +81 18 834 1111, Fax +81 18 836 2624

Fig. 1. CR3 expression on eosinophils with or without stimulation of PMA/ionomycin. Cells were stimulated by PMA 2.5 ng/ml and ionomycin 100 ng/ml (stimulation A), or PMA 25 ng/ml and ionomycin 1,000 ng/ml (stimulation B) for 45 min at 37 °C. Columns show mean values, and bars show SE.

Fig. 2. LFA1-α expression on eosinophils with or without stimulation of PMA/ionomycin. Cells were stimulated by PMA 2.5 ng/ml and ionomycin 100 ng/ml (stimulation A), or PMA 25 ng/ml and ionomycin 1,000 ng/ml (stimulation B) for 45 min at 37 °C. Columns show mean values, and bars show SE.

1

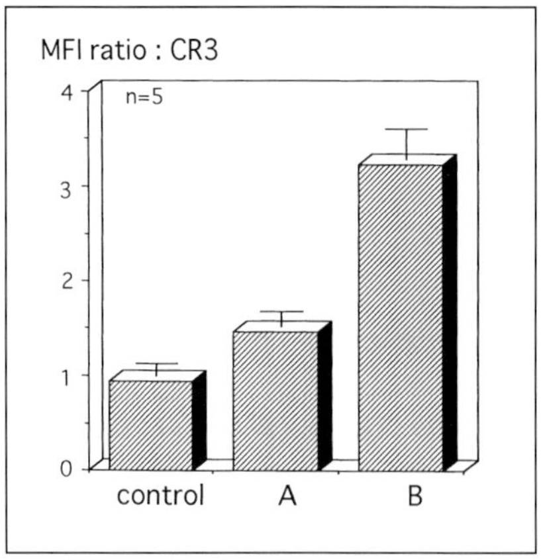

2

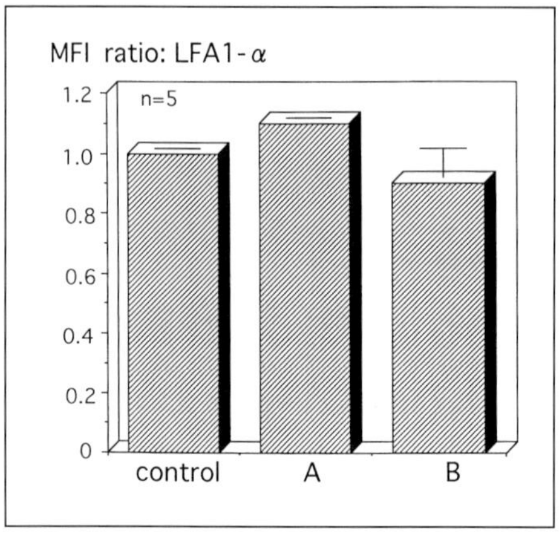

can damage bronchial mucosal cells, resulting in bronchial hyperresponsiveness [3]. Adhesion molecules may play an important role in allergic inflammation by activation of these cells (particularly eosinophils) [4, 5]. Therefore, the studies concerned with the mechanism of eosinophil activation may contribute to pathophysiological investigation of allergic disease. Such studies are associated with complications in isolating and purifying eosinophils. However, investigation of the activation of eosinophils has recently been performed by applying whole blood to a flow cytometer [6–8].

We investigated the usefulness of studying whole blood and labeling the EG2 antigen as an intracellular indicator for eosinophil activation and β_1 and β_2 integrin adhesion molecules as surface proteins [9]. In this study, we measured β_1, β_2 integrin quickly and conveniently with this method to evaluate eosinophil activation in vitro using phorbol-12-myristate-13-acetate (PMA)/ionomycin as stimulation.

Materials and Methods

After diluting 100 µl of heparinized whole blood with the same volume of RPMI 1640 (GIBCO, Grand Island, N.Y., USA), the samples were incubated with PMA (Sigma, St. Louis, Mo., USA) 2.5 ng/ml and ionomycin (Sigma) 100 ng/ml (as 'stimulation A'), or PMA 25 ng/ml and ionomycin 1,000 ng/ml (as 'stimulation B') for 45 min at 37 °C. Then, the cells were reacted with monoclonal antibody for adhesion molecules as follows: anti-human CR3-α chain (Nichirei, Tokyo), anti-human LFA1-α chain (Dako, Denmark), anti-human LFA1-β chain (Dako, Denmark), anti-human VLA-4-α chain (Immunotech, France) in the dark for 30 min at 4 °C and stained by FITC-conjugated secondary antibodies in the dark for 30 min at 4 °C. Then, 2 ml of the lysing solution (FACS™ Lysing Solution, Becton Dickinson, San Jose, Calif., USA) was added to each sample for hemolyzation of red blood cells. After centrifugation, the supernatant was discarded, and 100 µl of 0.4% *p*-benzoquinone (PBQ; Wako, Tokyo) was added, followed by incubation for 10 min in the dark at room temperature to fix the cells. Furthermore, the cells were treated with n-octyl-β-*D*-glucopyranoside (OG; Wako, Tokyo) to increase cell membrane permeability. The mean fluorescent intensity (MFI) was measured using flow cytometer (FACScan, Becton Dickinson) and the MFI ratio was calculated estimating MFI of each control at 1. All results were expressed as means ± SE, and significance was determined using the paired t test.

Results and Discussion

Although the evaluation of eosinophil activation in allergic inflammatory diseases, especially bronchial asthma, may provide useful information for pathophysiological studies, complications have been reported in isolating and purifying eosinophils. We investigated the usefulness of studying the eosinophil fraction in whole blood and labeling the EG2 antigen as an intracellular indicator for eosinophil activation [5, 6]. We found that whole blood analysis for characterizing eosinophils treated with PBQ and OG showed that EG2-positive eosinophils could easily be distinguished from other leukocyte fractions by gating in flow-cytometric analysis [7]. In this study, using this whole blood analysis, we measured β_2 and β_1 integrin on eosinophils stimulated by PMA/ionomycin to evaluate eosinophil activation in vitro. As shown in figure 1, when cells were stimulated with stimulation A or B of PMA/ionomycin for 45 min, both MFI ratios of CR3 were significantly higher than those of the unstimulated control. Concerning the MFI of the control at 1, the MFI ratio with stimulation A was 1.6 ± 0.1 ($p < 0.003$), the MFI ratio with stimulation B was 3.6 ± 0.4 ($p < 0.001$) and they showed a dose-dependent increase (fig. 1). However,

Fig. 3. LFA1-β expression on eosinophils with or without stimulation of PMA/ionomycin. Cells were stimulated by PMA 2.5 ng/ml and ionomycin 100 ng/ml (stimulation A), or PMA 25 ng/ml and ionomycin 1,000 ng/ml (stimulation B) for 45 min at 37 °C. Columns show mean values, and bars show SE.

Fig. 4. VLA-4 expression on eosinophils with or without stimulation of PMA/ionomycin. Cells were stimulated by PMA 2.5 ng/ml and ionomycin 100 ng/ml (stimulation A), or PMA 25 ng/ml and ionomycin 1,000 ng/ml (stimulation B) for 45 min at 37 °C. Columns show mean values, and bars show SE.

3

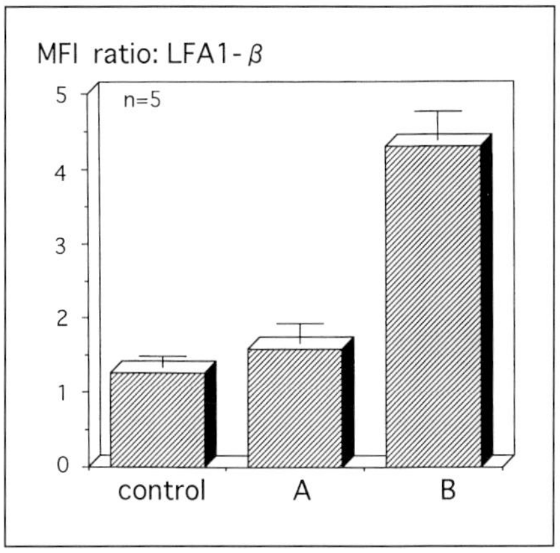

4

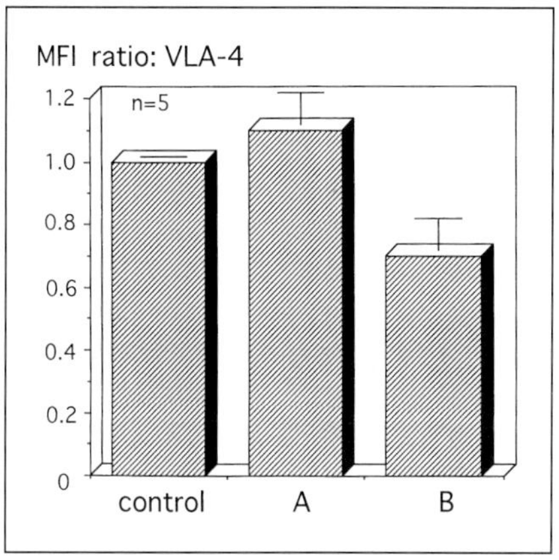

the MFI ratio of LFA1-α with stimulation A was 1.1 ± 0.048 ($p = 0.051$), the MFI ratio with stimulation B was 0.9 ± 0.1 ($p = 0.054$) and there were no significant differences compared to the unstimulated control (fig. 2). The MFI ratio of LFA1-β with stimulation A was 1.2 ± 0.1 ($p < 0.031$), the MFI ratio with stimulation B was 3.6 ± 0.4 ($p < 0.001$) and they revealed significant differences compared to the unstimulated control as well as a dose-dependent increase similar to CR3 (fig. 3). On the other hand, while the MFI ratio of VLA-4 with stimulation A was 1.1 ± 0.1 ($p < 0.324$) and there was no significant difference compared to the control, the MFI ratio with stimulation B was 0.7 ± 0.1 ($p < 0.001$) and a tendency to decrease was observed (fig. 4). The isolation and purification of eosinophils are time-consuming procedures in the preparation of experiments to study the properties of eosinophils. Our method of distinguishing eosinophils from various cell groups in whole blood, which is simple and time-saving, may allow intensive investigation of eosinophils in clinical laboratories as well as in research laboratories. The advantages of this whole blood analysis are as follows: (1) the procedure is simple and useful for healthy as well as hypereosinophilic subjects, (2) therefore, it is convenient to observe differences in reactions between asthmatic patients and healthy subjects especially those expected to reveal activation of eosinophils in vivo and (3) the reaction of eosinophils in this whole blood method may be more similar to reactions in vivo than those of purified eosinophils. We are currently investigating the influence of various kinds of stimulations, regulation factors or agents on eosinophils using this method.

References

1 Bousquet J, Chanez P, Lacoste JY, Barneon G, Chavanian N, Enancer I, Venge P, Ahlstedt S, Lafontaine JS, Godard P, Michel FB: Eosinophilic inflammation in asthma. N Engl J Med 1990;323:1033–1038.

2 Capron A, Ameisen JC, Joseph M, Auriault C, Tonnel AB, Caen J: New function for platelets and their pathological implications. Int Arch Allergy Appl Immunol 1985;77:107–114.

3 Gleich GJ, Adolphson CR: The eosinophilic leukocyte. Adv Immunol 1986;39:77–125.

4 Chihara J, Yamamoto T, Kurachi D, Nakajima S: Soluble ICAM-1 in sputum of patients with bronchial asthma. Lancet 1994;343:1108.

5 Chihara J, Kurachi D, Yamamoto T, Higashimoto I, Kakazu T, Nakajima S: Induction of β2 integrin expression on an eosinophilic cell line (EoL-1) by the supernatant of mononuclear cells stimulated with specific allergen from asthmatic patients. Immunol Lett 1994;42:25–29.

6 Krug N, Thurau M, Lackie P, Barier J, Scauer U: A flow cytometric method for the detection of intracellular basic proteins in unseparated peripheral blood and bone marrow eosinophils. J Immunol Methods 1996;190:245–254.

7 Hallden G, Anderson U, Hed J, Johansson SGO: A new membrane permeabilization method for the detection of intracellular antigens by flow cytometry. J Immunol Methods 1989;124:103–109.

8 Kuwasaki T, Chihara J, Kayaba H, Kamata Y, Oyamada H, Saito N, Shioya T, Sasaki M, Kagaya M, Tsuda A: Whole-blood flow-cytometric analysis of eosinophil EG2 expression as a marker of the pathological conditions of asthma. Int Arch Allergy Immunol 1998;117 (suppl 1):77–80.

9 Tai PC, Spry CJF, Peterson C, Venge P, Olsson I: Monoclonal antibodies distinguish between storage and secreted forms of eosinophil cationic protein. Nature 1984;309:182–184.

International Archives of
Allergy and
Immunology

Int Arch Allergy Immunol 1999;120(suppl 1):30–33

Interferon-γ Increases CD62L Expression on Human Eosinophils

T. Momose Y. Okubo S. Horie S. Takashi A. Tsukadaira J. Suzuki
M. Isobe M. Sekiguchi

First Department of Internal Medicine, Shinshu University School of Medicine, Matsumoto, Japan

Key Words
Eosinophils · CD62L · CD11b · Interferon-γ

Abstract
Background: L-selectin (CD62L) and Mac-1 (CD11b/CD18) play a crucial role in the infiltration of eosinophils. However, changes in CD62L and CD11b expression on eosinophils after stimulation with cytokines were little studied. ***Methods:*** Eosinophils in peripheral blood of healthy volunteers were purified and cultured with interleukin-5 (IL-5), granulocyte/macrophage colony-stimulating factor (GM-CSF) or interferon-γ (IFN-γ). After up to 24 h incubation, CD62L and CD11b expression were examined using flow cytometry. The effects of dexamethasone (Dex), cycloheximide (CHX) or theophylline on CD62L expression on IFN-γ-stimulated eosinophils were also studied. ***Results:*** IL-5 or GM-CSF downregulated CD62L and upregulated CD11b expression on eosinophils after 30 min stimulation. Conversely, IFN-γ upregulated CD62L after 12 h stimulation in a time- and dose-dependent manner, and had no effect on CD11b expression. Dex, CHX or theophylline dose-dependently decreased CD62L expression on IFN-γ-stimulated eosinophils. ***Conclusions:*** IFN-γ is a particular cytokine which can increase CD62L expression on circulating or infiltrated human eosinophils. It is suggested that protein synthesis and intracellular cAMP participate in the increase in L-selectin expression on IFN-γ-stimulated eosinophils.

Introduction

Infiltration of eosinophils to inflammatory foci is mediated by at least two classes of adhesion molecules [1, 2]. L-selectin (CD62L) is constitutively expressed on eosinophils, and plays an important role in the first step of extravasation. In sites of inflammation, circulating eosinophils roll on activated endothelial cells through binding of L-selectin to its ligands [3, 4]. Mac-1 (CD11b/CD18) is another adhesion molecule which mediates infiltration of eosinophils. Rapid shedding of L-selectin and concomitant increase of Mac-1 shift the cells from L-selectin-dependent rolling to Mac-1-dependent firm adhesion [5]. It has been reported that L-selectin is downregulated and Mac-1 is upregulated on infiltrated eosinophils in vivo [6, 7]. In addition to these adhesive functions, L-selectin and Mac-1 have signaling functions. L-selectin on neutrophils is involved in the increase of intracellular calcium, superoxide generation [8] and adhesive function via Mac-1 [9], and in the induction of mRNA for cytokines [10]. Mac-1

KARGER

Fax + 41 61 306 12 34
E-Mail karger@karger.ch
www.karger.com

1018–2438/99/1205–0030$17.50/0

Accessible online at:
http://BioMedNet.com/karger

Yoshio Okubo, MD
First Department of Internal Medicine, Shinshu University School of Medicine
3-1-1 Asahi
Matsumoto 390-8621 (Japan)
Tel. +81 263 35 4600, ext. 5252, Fax +81 263 36 3722

participates in granulocyte/macrophage colony-stimulating factor (GM-CSF)- or platelet-activating factor induced eosinophil degranulation [11], and cross-linking of Mac-1 as well as L-selectin induces a neutrophil superoxide generation [8]. Eosinophils are known to play an important role in the pathogenesis of late phase response and bronchial hyperresponsiveness in bronchial asthma [12]. The regulation of Mac-1 and L-selectin after eosinophil activation [5] and the inhibitory effect of a phosphodiesterase inhibitor [13] or a hydroxamate-based metalloprotease inhibitor [14] on the expression on these molecules are reported. Nevertheless, increase in CD62L expression on eosinophils have not been reported. In this study, we show that recombinant human (rh) interferon-γ (IFN-γ) upregulates CD62L expression on human eosinophils, in contrast to rh interleukin-5 (IL-5) and rhGM-CSF.

Material and Methods

Reagents

rhIL-5 was donated by Schering (Bloomfield, N.J., USA). rhGM-CSF and theophylline were provided by Kirin Brewery (Tokyo, Japan) and Otsuka Pharmaceutical Co. (Tokyo, Japan), respectively. rhIFN-γ was purchased from Genzyme (Cambridge, Mass., USA). Dexamethasone (Dex) and cycloheximide (CHX) were purchased from Sigma Chemical Co. (St. Louis, Mo., USA). Theophylline was dissolved in RPMI 1640 (Nikken Biological Laboratory, Kyoto, Japan) at 10^{-2} *M*. Dex and CHX were dissolved in dimethyl sulfoxide (Sigma) and in distilled water at 10^{-2} *M*, respectively, and stored at –20 °C.

Antibodies

Fluorescein isothiocyanate (FITC)-conjugated monoclonal antibody (mAb) against CD9 was purchased from Pharmingen (San Diego, Calif., USA). Phycoerythrin-conjugated anti-CD11b mAb and anti-CD62L mAb were purchased from DAKO Patts A/S (Grostrup, Denmark) and Becton Dickinson (San Jose, Calif., USA), respectively. Isotype-matched (mouse IgG1) FITC- and phycoerythrin-conjugated control mAbs were purchased from DAKO Patts A/S.

Eosinophil Purification

Eosinophil isolation was performed as previously reported [15]. Briefly, venous heparinized peripheral blood obtained from normal volunteers was mixed with 1 × piperazine-N,N-bis(2-ethanesulfonic acid) (PIPES) at a ratio of 1:1. The diluted blood was overlayered on Percoll solution (density 1.082; Sigma) and centrifuged at 1,000 *g* for 30 min at 4 °C. The mononuclear cell layer was then carefully removed and erythrocytes were lysed by two cycles of hypotonic shock with distilled water. The isolated granulocytes were washed twice with PIPES buffer supplemented with 1% inactivated fetal calf serum (FCS; Life Technologies, Gaithersburg, Md., USA). The resultant pellet of granulocytes was incubated with anti-CD16 mAb conjugated with immunomagnetic particles (Miltenyi Biotec, Bergisch-Gladbach, Germany; 50 µl for 5 × 10^7 cells) for 1 h on ice. Magnetically labeled neutrophils were then depleted by passage through a magnetic cell separation column in the field of permanent magnet (Miltenyi Biotec). This procedure results in more than 98% pure eosinophils with >99% viability.

Cell Culture and Flow Cytometry

The purified eosinophils were suspended at 1 × 10^6 cells/ml in RPMI 1640 supplemented with 10% FCS and 50 µg/ml gentamycin. The cell suspension (1 ml) was added to each well of a culture plate (Falcon No. 3047, Becton Dickinson, San Jose, Calif., USA). The cytokines (rhIL-5 100 pg/ml, rhGM-CSF 1 ng/ml, rhIFN-γ 0.1–100 U/ml) and the drugs (theophylline 10^{-5} to 10^{-3} *M*, CHX 10^{-8} to 10^{-6} *M*, Dex 10^{-8} to 10^{-6} *M*) were then added to certain wells, and cell culture was performed at 37 °C in a humid atmosphere with 5% CO_2. After incubation, the cells were collected and washed twice with 1 × PIPES containing 1% FCS. Subsequently, the cells were reacted with each mAb (anti-CD9, anti-CD62L, anti-CD11b and control Ab) at 4 °C for 30 min. CD62L and CD11b expression was then examined with FACScan (Becton Dickinson). Eosinophils were gated using combined forward and side light scattering and confirmed with FITC-conjugated anti-CD9 mAb. Data were collected on 1 × 10^4 gated cells per sample and analyzed using the Consort 32 program (Becton Dickinson) [16]. The changes of mean fluorescence intensity (MFI) of adhesion molecules by stimulators or drugs were calculated as follows:

% increase = [(MFI of stimulated cells – MFI of cultured cells without stimuli) / MFI of fresh cells] × 100

Statistical Analysis

Data are expressed as mean ± SEM. Basic statistical evaluation was performed using one-way ANOVA; Fisher's PLSD method was employed when significant ($p < 0.05$) statistical results were noted.

Results

rhIL-5 (100 pg/ml) or rhGM-CSF (1 ng/ml) downregulated CD62L and upregulated CD11b expression on human eosinophils after 4 h stimulation (table 1). In contrast, rhIFN-γ (0.1–100 U/ml) increased CD62L expression after 12 h stimulation in a dose-dependent manner, and had no significant effect on CD11b expression (table 1). Theophylline (a phosphodiesterase inhibitor that increases intracellular cAMP), Dex or CHX (inhibitors against protein synthesis) decreased MFI of CD62L on rhIFN-γ-stimulated eosinophils in a dose-dependent fashion (table 2). Furthermore, effects of tumor necrosis factor-α (10 ng/ml), platelet-activating factor (10^{-6} *M*), eotaxin (10 ng/ml), RANTES (100 ng/ml) or monocyte chemoattractant protein-3 (100 ng/ml) on CD62L and CD11b expression on human eosinophils were similar to those of rhIL-5 and rhGM-CSF (data not shown).

Table 1. Changes in CD62L and CD11b expression

	n	Increase, %		
		4 h	12 h	24 h
CD62L				
rhIL-5: 100 pg/ml	3	−73.3 ± 8.1*	−54.7 ± 4.6*	−67.0 ± 4.8*
rhGM-CSF: 1 ng/ml	3	−44.8 ± 9.9*	−26.5 ± 4.4*	−22.5 ± 2.4*
rhIFN-γ				
0.1 U/ml	3	2.0 ± 4.4	0.7 ± 0.5	12.2 ± 9.0
1 U/ml	3	4.3 ± 1.6	7.7 ± 0.2	20.2 ± 2.9
10 U/ml	3	3.7 ± 2.8	17.9 ± 3.8*	43.5 ± 7.8*
100 U/ml	4	2.3 ± 1.5	17.9 ± 4.1*	52.2 ± 10.7*
CD11b				
rhIL-5: 100 pg/ml	3	62.3 ± 5.4*	25.0 ± 3.0*	22.4 ± 2.7*
rhGM-CSF: 1 ng/ml	3	63.0 ± 3.4*	26.6 ± 2.6*	21.2 ± 2.7*
rhIFN-γ: 100 U/ml	4	1.6 ± 3.1	1.1 ± 2.0	3.4 ± 1.8

Increase was calculated as described in Material and Methods. * $p < 0.05$ vs. 0%. n = Number of experiments.

Table 2. Effects of CHX and Dex

		n	Increase, %
Control		3	53.6 ± 6.4
Dex	10^{-6} *M*	3	10.5 ± 1.1*
	10^{-7} *M*	3	15.0 ± 0.6*
	10^{-8} *M*	3	36.0 ± 2.2*
CHX	10^{-6} *M*	3	12.2 ± 1.9*
	10^{-7} *M*	3	39.0 ± 3.1*
	10^{-8} *M*	3	48.5 ± 3.9

Eosinophils were incubated for 24 h with 100 U/ml rhIFN-γ. * $p < 0.05$ vs. control. n = Number of experiments.

Discussion

In this study, we demonstrated that rhIFN-γ increases CD62L expression on human eosinophils in contrast to other eosinophil activators, and that intracellular cAMP and protein synthesis may be involved in CD62L upregulation on rhIFN-γ-stimulated eosinophils. Our results indicate that rhIFN-γ is a particular cytokine which can increase CD62L expression on circulating or infiltrated eosinophils. Iwamoto et al. [17] reported that recombinant IFN-γ reduces antigen-induced eosinophil recruitment into the mouse airways; they attributed the inhibitory effect of IFN-γ to the reduction of CD4+ T cell infiltration. The increase in CD62L expression on circulating eosinophils may be another possible mechanism of reduced eosinophil recruitment, because a shift from L-selectin-dependent rolling to Mac-1-dependent adhesion is an important step for extravasation [5]. Although it has been reported that CD62L on neutrophils participates in certain neutrophil functions [8–10], little is known about the signaling function of CD62L on eosinophils. IFN-γ is detected in the serum of asthmatics [18]; increased CD62L by IFN-γ may play a role in certain eosinophil biological functions. The presented results suggest that further studies on the function of CD62L on infiltrated eosinophils are warranted.

References

1 Kishimoto TK, Jutila MA, Berg EL, Butcher EC: Neutrophil Mac-1 and MEL-14 adhesion proteins inversely regulated by chemotactic factors. Science 1989;245:1238–1241.

2 Bochner BS, Schleimer RP: The role of adhesion molecules in human eosinophil and basophil recruitment. J Allergy Clin Immunol 1994; 94:427–438.

3 Sriramarao P, von Andrian UH, Butcher EC, Bourdon MA, Broide DH: L-selectin and very late antigen-4 integrin promote eosinophil rolling at physiological shear rates in vivo. J Immunol 1994;153:4238–4246.

4 Knol EF, Tackey F, Tedder TF, Klunk DA, Bickel CA, Sterbinsky SA, Bochner BS: Comparison of human eosinophil and neutrophil adhesion to endothelial cells under nonstatic conditions. Role of L-selectin. J Immunol 1994;153:2161–2167.

5 Neeley SP, Hamann KJ, White SR, Baranowski SL, Burch RA, Leff AR: Selective regulation of expression of surface adhesion molecules Mac-1, L-selectin, and VLA-4 on human eosinophils and neutrophils. Am J Respir Cell Mol Biol 1993;8:633–639.

6 Mengelers HJ, Maikoe T, Hooibrink B, Kuypers TW, Kreukniet J, Lammers JW, Koenderman L: Down modulation of L-selectin expression on eosinophils recovered from bronchoalveolar lavage fluid after allergen provocation. Clin Exp Allergy 1993;23:196–204.

7 Georas SN, Liu MC, Newman W, Beall LD, Stealey BA, Bochner BS: Altered adhesion molecule expression and endothelial cell activation accompany the recruitment of human granulocytes to the lung after segmental antigen challenge. Am J Respir Cell Mol Biol 1992;7:261–269.

8 Crockett-Torabi E, Sulenbarger B, Smith CW, Fantone JC: Activation of human neutrophils through L-selectin and Mac-1 molecules. J Immunol 1995;154:2291–2302.
9 Simon SI, Burns AR, Taylor AD, Gopalan PK, Lynam EB, Sklar LA, Smith CW: L-selectin (CD62L) cross-linking signals neutrophil adhesive functions via the Mac-1 (CD11b/CD18) beta 2-integrin. J Immunol 1995;155:1502–1514.
10 Laudanna C, Constantin G, Baron P, Scarpini E, Scarlato G, Cabrini G, Dechecchi C, Rossi F, Cassatella MA, Berton G: Sulfatides trigger increase of cytosolic free calcium and enhanced expression of tumor necrosis factor-alpha and interleukin-8 mRNA in human neutrophils. Evidence for a role of L-selectin as a signaling molecule. J Biol Chem 1994;269:4021–4026.
11 Horie S, Kita H: CD11b/CD18 (Mac-1) is required for degranulation of human eosinophils induced by human recombinant granulocyte-macrophage colony-stimulating factor and platelet-activating factor. J Immunol 1994;152:5457–5467.
12 Frigas E, Gleich GJ: The eosinophil and pathophysiology of asthma. J Allergy Clin Immunol 1986;77:527–537.
13 Berends C, Dijkhuizen B, de Monchy JG, Dubois AE, Gerritsen J, Kauffman HF: Inhibition of PAF-induced expression of CD11b and shedding of L-selectin on human neutrophils and eosinophils by the type IV selective PDE inhibitor, rolipram. Eur Respir J 1997;10:1000–1007.
14 Bennett TA, Lynam EB, Sklar LA, Rojelj S: Hydroxamate-based metalloprotease inhibitor blocks shedding of L-selectin adhesion molecule from leukocytes: Functional consequences for neutrophil aggregation. J Immunol 1996;156:3093–3097.
15 Hossain M, Okubo Y, Horie S, Sekiguchi M: Analysis of recombinant human tumour necrosis factor-alpha-induced CD4 expression on human eosinophils. Immunology 1996;88:301–307.
16 Okubo Y, Hossain M, Kai R, Sato E, Honda T, Sekiguchi M, Itoh S, Takatsu K: Adhesion molecules on eosinophils in acute eosinophilic pneumonia. Am J Respir Crit Care Med 1995;151:1259–1262.
17 Iwamoto I, Nakajima H, Endo H, Yoshida S: Interferon gamma regulates antigen-induced eosinophil recruitment into the mouse airways by inhibiting the infiltration of CD4+ T cells. J Exp Med 1993;177:573–576.
18 Saito H, Hayakawa T, Mita H, Yui Y, Shida T: Augmentation of leukotriene C4 production by gamma interferon in leukocytes challenged with antigen. Int Arch Allergy Appl Immunol 1988;87:286–293.

International Archives of
Allergy and Immunology

Int Arch Allergy Immunol 1999;120(suppl 1):34–37

Adhesion to Fibronectin Regulates Expression of Intercellular Adhesion Molecule-1 on Eosinophilic Cells

Ikkou Higashimoto[a] Junichi Chihara[b] Masaharu Kawabata[a]
Shigenori Nakajima[c] Mitsuhiro Osame[a]

[a]Third Department of Internal Medicine, Kagoshima University Faculty of Medicine, Kagoshima,
[b]Department of Clinical and Laboratory Medicine, Akita University School of Medicine, Akita, and
[c]Fourth Department of Internal Medicine, Kinki University School of Medicine, Osaka, Japan

Key Words
Adhesion molecules · Eosinophil · Fibronectin · ICAM-1 · VLA-4

Abstract
Background: Adhesion molecules may play an important role in eosinophilic activation as well as adherence of extracellular matrix (ECM) including fibronectin (FN) in the inflamed focus. Tissue eosinophils expressed intercellular adhesion molecule-1 (ICAM-1, CD54), whereas peripheral blood eosinophils did not. The molecular mechanisms of ICAM-1 expression on eosinophils are not clear. We immunologically examined the effect of adherence to FN on the expression of adhesion molecules in an eosinophilic cell line (EoL-1). ***Methods:*** EoL-1 cells, suspended at a concentration of 2×10^6 cells/ml, were cultured at 37 °C in BSA or FN-coated 24-well plates. After 4 h, the cells were removed by pipetting, and the expression of adhesion molecules was evaluated by immunofluorescence. ***Results:*** Adherence of EoL-1 to FN enhanced ICAM-1 (CD54) expression on EoL-1 (FN vs. BSA: 84.76 ± 17.90 vs. 43.73 ± 7.60, mean fluorescent intensity). Regarding other adhesion molecules on EoL-1 (CD11a, CD18, CD49d), the expression was not significantly augmented by adherence to FN. ***Conclusions:*** We concluded that the signal via adhesion of FN regulates the expression of ICAM-1 on eosinophilic cells. This study suggests that eosinophilic adhesion to ECM via adhesion molecules plays an important role in the pathogenesis of allergic inflammation through eosinophilic functional changes, including regulation of expressive adhesion molecules such as ICAM-1.

Introduction

Eosinophils are major inflammatory effector cells with blood and tissue eosinophilia being a feature of many allergic disorders, such as bronchial asthma [1–4]. Recently, adhesion molecules have been considered to play an important role in eosinophilic activation as well as adherence of extracellular matrix (ECM) including fibronectin (FN) in the inflamed focus. Therefore, it is of interest to evaluate eosinophilic activation via signals by adherence of eosinophils to ECM. The signal via adhesion molecules regulates the function of the eosinophilic cell line, EoL-1 [5, 6].

KARGER
Fax + 41 61 306 12 34
E-Mail karger@karger.ch
www.karger.com

1018–2438/99/1205–0034$17.50/0

Accessible online at:
http://BioMedNet.com/karger

Ikkou Higashimoto, MD
Third Department of Internal Medicine
Kagoshima University Faculty of Medicine
Kagoshima 890 (Japan)
Tel. +81 99 275 5332, Fax +81 99 265 7164

Furthermore, tissue eosinophils were found to express intercellular adhesion molecule-1 (ICAM-1, CD54), whereas peripheral blood eosinophils did not [7, 8]. We previously revealed a high expression of ICAM-1 on hypodense eosinophils, which are activated eosinophils [9]. Thus, in this study, to evaluate eosinophilic activation in adhesion molecule expression via FN signals, we examined the effect of adhesion to FN, which belongs to the ECM, on expressive adhesion molecules in eosinophilic cells.

Materials and Methods

Reagents

Human plasma fibronectin was obtained from Wako Pure Chemicals (Osaka, Japan). Monoclonal antibodies (mAbs) used were MHM24 (anti-CD11a) and MHM23 (anti-CD18) obtained from Dako (Denmark), OKM-1 (anti-CD11b) obtained from Ortho Diagnostic Systems (Westwood, Mass., USA) and HP2/1 (anti-CDw49d) and 84H10 (anti-CD54) obtained from Immunotech (France).

Cell Line and Culture Conditions

EoL-1 cells, established from the peripheral blood of a patient with eosinophilic leukemia, were suspended at a concentration of 2×10^6 cells/ml in RPMI-1640 with 5% fetal calf serum (M.A. Bioproducts) and antibiotics (100 μg/ml penicillin and 100 μg/ml streptomycin). Cells were cultured at 37 °C in a humidified 5% CO_2 atmosphere in BSA or FN-coated 24-well plates (Falcon; Becton-Dickinson, Mountain View, Calif., USA). Three hundred microliters of FN (100 μg/ml in PBS) or BSA (100 μg/ml in PBS) was added to each well for 1 h at 37 °C. The plates were then washed twice with PBS to remove unbound protein. To block nonspecific protein-binding sites, 200 μl of 1% heat-denatured BSA in PBS was added to each well, and the plates were incubated for 2 h at room temperature. Before cells were added, the plates were washed twice with RPMI/1% BSA. After 4 h, the cells were removed by pipetting, and the expression of adhesion molecules was evaluated by immunofluorescence.

Surface Marker Analysis of EoL-1

Surface markers were examined by indirect immunofluorescent studies. Briefly, cells (50 μl, 5×10^6/ml) were incubated for 45 min at 4 °C with the specific mAb or control antibody. mAbs were used at a final concentration of 10 μg/ml. Cells were then washed and incubated for an additional 45 min at 4 °C with a FITC-conjugated goat anti-mouse IgG antibody (Tago, Burlingame, Calif., USA). After 2 washings, quantitative analysis of the stained cells was performed using a FACScan (Becton-Dickinson). The mean fluorescent intensity (MFI) was determined from at least 10,000 counted cells.

Statistical Analysis

Data were expressed as means ± SE. Statistical analysis was performed using Student's t test. A p value of <0.05 was considered to indicate statistical significance.

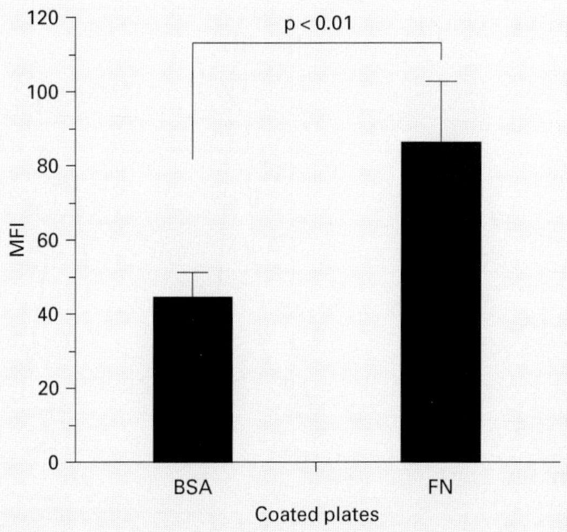

Fig. 1. Comparison of ICAM-1 (CD54) expression on eosinophils incubated on BSA- and FN-coated plates for 4 h. Values are the MFI (mean ± SE) from 9 independent experiments.

Results

Adherence to FN enhanced ICAM-1 (CD54) expression on EoL-1 compared to that to BSA as a control (fig. 1). MFI, as an expression of ICAM-1 on EoL-1 cultured in FN-coated plates for 4 h, was 84.71 ± 17.90, while that in BSA-coated plates was 43.73 ± 7.40 ($p < 0.01$). Regarding other adhesion molecules on EoL-1 (CD11a, CD18, CD49d), the expression was not significantly augmented by adherence to FN (fig. 2).

Discussion

Eosinophils are important effector cells in allergic inflammatory diseases such as bronchial asthma [1, 2]. In addition, adhesion molecules play an important role in the accumulation of eosinophils in inflamed sites [10].

Although the molecular mechanisms of eosinophilic recruitment remain unclear, VLA-4, a β_1 integrin molecule expressed on eosinophils but not on neutrophils, may selectively recruit eosinophils to inflamed airway tissue in bronchial asthma such as allergic inflammation [11, 12]. The ligand for VLA-4 is VCAM-1, which is expressed on endothelium and fibronectin, and belongs to the extracellular matrix in the interstitium.

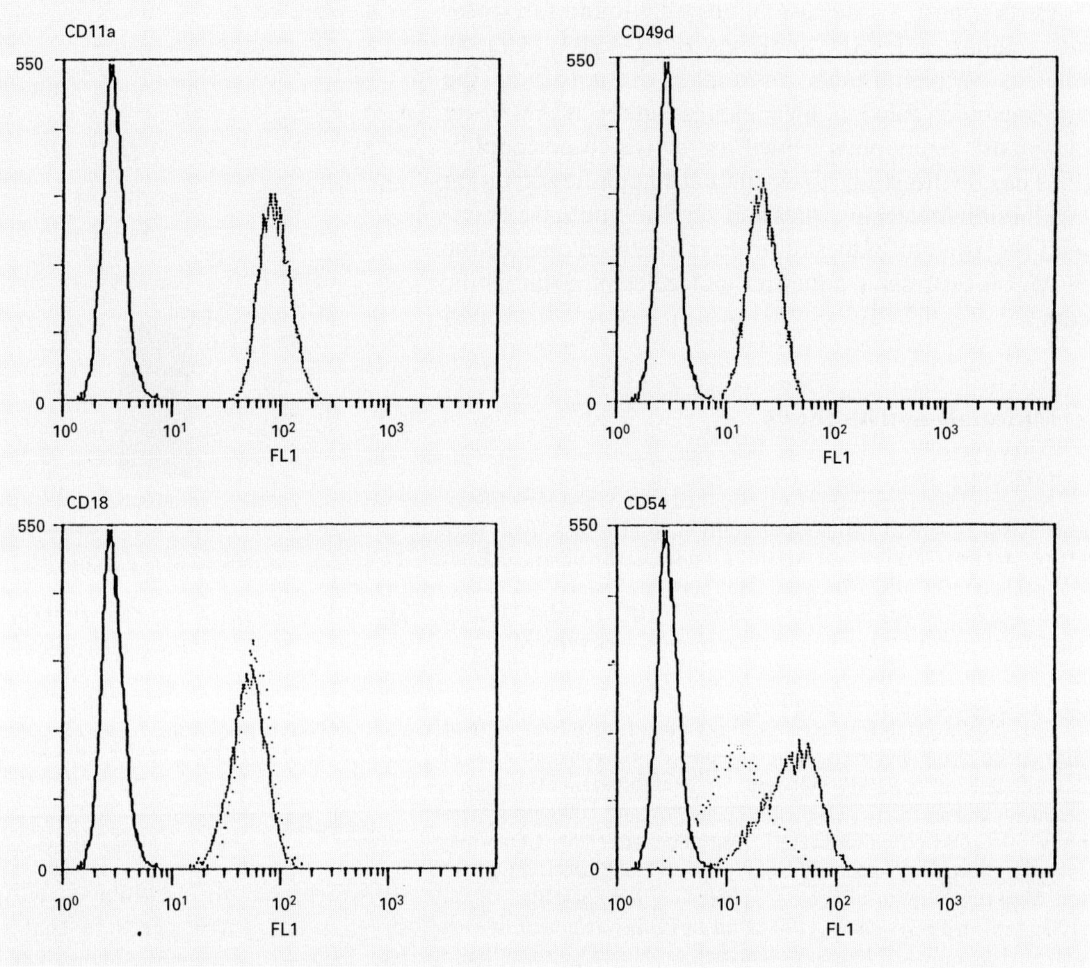

Fig. 2. Histograms show logarithmic mean fluorescence frequency distribution analysis of 10,000 EoL-1 cells stained for adhesion molecules (CD11a, CD18, CD49d, CD54) cultured on BSA (······)- or FN (– – –)-coated plates, with control isotype-matched mouse IgG (——) for 4 h.

Expression of adhesion molecules on eosinophils is inducible or modulated by various stimuli [13, 14]. IL-3, IL-5 [15], GM-CSF and chemokine RANTES [16] are involved in CD11b expression on eosinophils.

ICAM-1 expression on eosinophils may have important implications for eosinophilic function in cell networks, interaction with other eosinophils, T cells and macrophages via LFA-1 molecules [17, 18]. Recent studies showed that higher levels of ICAM-1 molecules were expressed on eosinophils which were accumulated in bronchial tissues [7, 8, 19] and sputum from asthmatic subjects [20, 21], or obtained from peripheral blood of hypereosinophilic patients [9]. The upregulation could be induced by soluble stimuli of TNF-α and other cytokines [22, 23]. In addition to the involvement of cytokines, we demonstrated here that the interaction with FN via the VLA-4 molecule regulates the expression of another adhesion molecule, ICAM-1, on eosinophilic cell lines.

In this study, ICAM-1 expression on cells with FN was significantly enhanced compared with that on BSA-coated plates. To investigate whether or not the underlying mechanism is specifically mediated by VLA-4 molecules, according to our preliminary examination, similar results were induced by specific bindings of VLA-4 using anti-CDw49d antibody (HP2/1; data not shown).

Recently, Anwar et al. [24] reported that adhesion to FN prolongs survival of eosinophils in culture by triggering autocrine generation of cytokines, IL-3 and GM-CSF. On the other hand, we previously reported that β_2 integrin (CD11a, CD11b, CD18) expression on EoL-1 was upregulated by the supernatant of mononuclear cells stimulated with specific allergens from asthmatic subjects [25]. We observed that the cytokines of IL-3, GM-CSF and IL-5 also enhanced these β_2 integrins. However, the absence of changes in the β_2 integrin expression on EoL-1 induced by adhesion to FN in the present study suggested that the mechanism is not mediated by these cytokines. When EoL-1 was incubated on FN with mAbs (anti-IL-3, anti-IL-5, anti-GM-CSF), enhancement of ICAM-1 expression was only partially inhibited (data not shown). We speculated that the induction mechanism of ICAM-1 expression of EoL-1 is mediated by direct intracellular transduction of activation of signals or other cytokines.

In summary, we demonstrated that eosinophilic interaction with FN induces the augmentative effect of ICAM-1 expression on EoL-1. Thus, we concluded that signals via cell adherence by adhesion molecules play an important role in the cell-cell interactive pathogenesis of allergic inflammation through involvement of eosinophilic functions in adhesion molecule expression.

Acknowledgment

We thank Drs. T. Kakazu, T. Yamamoto, D. Kurachi, and N.H. Kameda for their support and helpful discussions.

References

1 Bousquet J, Chanez P, Lacoste JY, et al: Eosinophilic inflammation in asthma. N Engl J Med 1990;323:1033–1039.
2 Gleich GJ, Adolphson CR: The eosinophil leukocyte: Structure and function. Adv Immunol 1986;39:177–253.
3 Carlos TM, Harlan JM: Leukocyte-endothelial adhesion molecules. Blood 1994;84:2068–2101.
4 Butcher EC: Leukocyte-endothelial cell recognition: Three (or more) steps to specificity and diversity. Cell 1991;67:1033–1036.
5 Saito H, Bourinbaiar A, Ginsburg M, Minato K, Ceresi E, Yamada K, Machover D, Breard J, Mathe G: Establishment and characterization of a new human eosinophilic leukemia cell line. Blood 1985;66:1233–1240.
6 Morita M, Saito H: Differentiation of a human eosinophilic cell line (EoL-1) by a human T-cell leukemia cell line (HHIL-3)-derived factor. Blood 1991;77:1766–1775.
7 Bentley AM, Durham SR, Robinson SD, Menz G, Storz C, Cromwell O, Kay AB, Wardlaw AJ: Expression of endothelial and leukocyte adhesion molecules intercellular adhesion molecule-1, E-selectin, and vascular cell adhesion molecule-1 in the bronchial mucosa in steady-state and allergic-induced asthma. J Allergy Clin Immunol 1993;92:857–868.
8 Sedgwick JB, Calhoun WJ, Vrtis RF, Bates ME, McAllister PK, Busse WW: Comparison of airway and blood eosinophil function after in vivo antigen challenge. J Immunol 1992; 149:3710–3718.
9 Chihara J, Yasukawa A, Yamamoto T, Kurachi D, Nakajima S: Characteristics of adhesion molecules expression on eosinophils with hypereosinophilia. Allergy Clin Immunol News 1991;(suppl 1):144.
10 Wegener CD, Gundel RH, Reilly P, Haynes N, Letts LG, Rothlein R: Intercellular adhesion molecule-1 (ICAM-1) in the pathogenesis of asthma. Science 1990;247:456–459.
11 Bochner BS, Luscinskas FW, Gimbrone MA Jr, Newman W, Sterbinsky SA, Derse-Anthony CP, Klunk D, Schleimer RP: Adhesion of human basophils, eosinophils, and neutrophils to interleukin 1-activated human vascular endothelial cells: Contributions of endothelial cell adhesion molecules. J Exp Med 1991;173: 1553–1556.
12 Walsh GM, Mermod JJ, Hartnell A, Kay AB, Wardlaw AJ: Human eosinophil, but not neutrophil, adherence to IL-1-stimulated human umbilical vascular endothelial cells is $\alpha_4\beta_1$ (very late antigen-4) dependent. J Immunol 1991;146:3419–3423.
13 Ebisawa M, Bochner BS, Georas SN, Schleimer RP: Eosinophil transendothelial migration induced by cytokines. J Immunol 1992;149: 4021–4028.
14 Walker C, Rifs S, Braun RK, Betz S, Bruijnzeel PLB: Increased expression of CD11b and functional changes in eosinophils after migration across endothelial cell monolayers. J Immunol 1993;150:4061–4071.
15 Walsh GM, Hartnell A, Wardlaw AJ, Kurihara K, Sanderson CJ, Kay AB: IL-5 enhances the in vitro adhesion of human eosinophils, but not neutrophils, in a leukocyte integrin (CD11/CD18)-dependent manner. Immunology 1990; 71:258–265.
16 Alam R, Stafford S, Forsythe P, Bogue DT, Harrison R, Faubion D, Lett-Brown MA, Grant JA: RANTES is a chemotactic and activating factor for human eosinophil. J Immunol 1993;150:3442–3447.
17 Oppenheimer-Marks N, Davis LS, Bogue DT, Ramberg J, Lipsky PE: Differential utilization of ICAM-1 and VCAM-1 during the adhesion and transendothelial migration of human T lymphocytes. J Immunol 1991;147:2913–2921.
18 Horie S, Okubo Y, Hossain M, Momose T, Suzuki J, Isobe M, Sekiguchi M: Intercellular adhesion molecule-1 on eosinophils is involved in eosinophil protein X release induced by cytokines. Immunology 1997;90(2):301–307.
19 Hansel TT, Walker C: The migration of eosinophils into the sputum of asthmatics: The role of adhesion molecules. Clin Exp Allergy 1992;22: 345–356.
20 Hansel TT, Braunstein JB, Walker C, Blaser K, Bruijnzeel PL, Virchow JC Jr, Virchow C Sr: Sputum eosinophils from asthmatics express ICAM-1 and HLA-DR. Clin Exp Immunol 1991;86:271–277.
21 Louis R, Shute J, Stanciu L, Marrelli F, Tetor H, Hidi R, Djukanovic R: Cell infiltration, ICAM-1 expression, and eosinophil chemotactic activity in asthmatic sputum. Am J Respir Crit Care Med 1997;155(2):466–472.
22 Hansel TT, De-Vries IJM, Carballido JM, Braun RK, Carballido-Perrig N, Rihs S, Blaser K, Walker C: Induction and function of eosinophil intercellular adhesion molecule-1 and HLA-DR. J Immunol 1992;149:2130–2136.
23 Georas SN, Liu MC, Newman W, Beall LD, Stealey BA, Bochner BS: Altered adhesion molecule expression and endothelial cell activation accompany the recruitment of human granulocytes to the lung after segmental antigen challenge. Am J Respir Cell Mol Biol 1992;7:261–269.
24 Anwar ARF, Moqbel R, Walsh GM, Kay AB, Wardlaw AJ: Adhesion to fibronectin prolongs eosinophil survival. J Exp Med 1993;177:839–843.
25 Chihara J, Kurachi D, Yamamoto T, Higashimoto I, Kakazu T, Nakajima S: Induction of β_2 integrin expression on an eosinophilic cell line (EoL-1) by the supernatant of mononuclear cells stimulated with specific allergen from asthmatic patients. Immunol Lett 1994;42:25–29.

International Archives of Allergy and Immunology

Int Arch Allergy Immunol 1999;120(suppl 1):38–44

Functional Expression of Transmembrane 4 Superfamily Molecules on Human Eosinophils

Kenji Matsumoto[a,b] Bruce S. Bochner[b] Hiroshi Wakiguchi[a] Takanobu Kurashige[a]

[a]Department of Pediatrics, Kochi Medical School, Nankoku City, Kochi, Japan;
[b]Division of Allergy and Clinical Immunology, Johns Hopkins Asthma and Allergy Center, Baltimore, Md., USA

Key Words

Eosinophil · Transmembrane 4 superfamily · CD9 · CD37 · CD53 · CD63 · CD81 · Homotypic aggregation · CD11b · CD62L

Abstract

Background: Transmembrane 4 superfamily (TM4SF) molecules are exclusively found on hematopoietic cells. Several members of the TM4SF are reported to be associated with other cell surface molecules, including integrins, and might participate in signal transduction, but little is known about their role on eosinophils. In the present study, we determined the expression and function of TM4SF molecules on human eosinophils. ***Methods:*** Surface expression of TM4SF molecules on purified peripheral blood eosinophils was examined using indirect immunofluorescence and flow cytometry. Purified eosinophils were incubated with anti-TM4SF monoclonal antibodies (mAbs) for up to 24 h. Eosinophil activation was evaluated by measuring eosinophil homotypic aggregation as well as changes in surface expression of CD11b or CD62L by flow cytometry. ***Results:*** Freshly isolated eosinophils expressed CD9, CD37, CD53, CD63 and CD81. Incubation with anti-CD9 mAb but not with anti-CD37, CD53, CD63 or CD81 mAb induced significant eosinophil homotypic aggregation. Incubation with any of the anti-TM4SF mAb for 30 min failed to alter the expression of either CD11b or CD62L on eosinophils. In contrast, the expression of CD11b was significantly enhanced after 24 h of incubation with anti-CD53 mAb, while the expression of CD62L was significantly reduced with anti-CD81 mAb. ***Conclusions:*** Cross-linking of some surface TM4SF molecules induced significant eosinophil homotypic aggregation, upregulation of CD11b expression, or CD62L shedding, consistent with activation of eosinophils. Our data suggest that several TM4SF molecules are functionally expressed on human eosinophils, and therefore might participate in allergic inflammation.

Introduction

Eosinophils are known to be important effector cells in helminth infections and allergic diseases [1]. Not only eosinophil-activating cytokines such as IL-3, IL-5 and granulocyte-macrophage colony-stimulating factor (GM-CSF) [2], as well as several eosinophil surface molecules, including adhesion molecules, are capable of modulating eosinophil functions [3]. Eosinophils express a wide variety of adhesion molecules that allow them to interact with

KARGER

Fax +41 61 306 12 34
E-Mail karger@karger.ch
www.karger.com

Accessible online at:
http://BioMedNet.com/karger

Dr. Kenji Matsumoto
Department of Pediatrics, Kochi Medical School
Kohasu, Okoh-Chou, Nankoku City, Kochi, 783-8505 (Japan)
Tel. +81 888 80 2355, Fax +81 888 80 2356
E-Mail yuiiku@med.kochi-ms.ac.jp

other cells and with extracellular matrix proteins [4]. Among them, integrins play a central role in eosinophil activation in allergic inflammation [5]. For instance, CD49d/CD29, a β_1 integrin heterodimer (VLA-4), plays a key role in selective eosinophil infiltration into allergic inflammatory sites [6], induces superoxide generation [7], and promotes eosinophil survival by activating GM-CSF autocrine pathway [8, 9]. Another integrin heterodimer, CD11b/CD18, a β_2 integrin heterodimer (Mac-1) plays a crucial role in eosinophil degranulation [10]. As far as signal transduction pathways through integrins are concerned, several molecules cluster to form a so-called integrin complex [11], which can transduce activation signals upon aggregation. Activation signals are mediated not through the integrins themselves but through other clustered structures which undergo phosphorylation of tyrosine residues by several kinases [12]. We have shown that eosinophil activation was found upon ligation of CD45 isoforms, another functionally associated molecule for integrin on eosinophils [13].

The transmembrane 4 superfamily (TM4SF) comprises a group of cell surface proteins including CD9, CD37, CD53, CD63 and CD81, which are characterized by the presence of four hydrophobic domains spanning the cell membrane [14]. Recently, association of several TM4SF molecules in integrin complexes has been reported. For example, molecules including CD9, CD53, CD63 and CD81 have been detected in association with integrin $\alpha_4\beta_1$ (CD49d/CD29) [15–17]. Other examples include the association of CD9 with CD29, CD49b, CD49c, CD49f, CD51/61 and HLA-DR; CD37 with CD53, CD81 and MHC class II; CD53 with CD20, CD81, MHC class I, MHC class II and HLA-DR; CD63 with CD49c, CD49e, CD29, CD11 and CD18 [18], and CD81 with CD19, CD20, CD21, CD53 and HLA-DR [19].

The conserved structure of TM4SF molecules suggests that they might work as part of a receptor complex or as a receptor itself. To date, no direct ligand for TM4SF molecules has been identified. However, several monoclonal antibodies (mAbs) against TM4SF molecules are capable of activating some types of inflammatory cells. In lymphocytes, functional studies of TM4SF molecules have been well studied, but little is known about TM4SF molecules on granulocytes. In eosinophils, we have only one information showing that immobilized but not soluble mAb against CD9 induces eosinophil degranulation and prolongs eosinophil survival by activating the GM-CSF autocrine pathway [20].

As TM4SF molecules are reported to be physiologically or functionally associated with several molecules present on eosinophils, especially integrins [19, 21], we hypothesized that TM4SF molecules might be involved in eosinophil activation and might be a target for selective regulation of allergic inflammation. To examine the function and expression of TM4SF molecules on eosinophils, we assessed the expression of several members of TM4SF molecules on human peripheral blood eosinophils and cultured them in the presence of anti-TM4SF mAbs. In the present study, eosinophil activation was assessed in three different ways by analyzing eosinophil homotypic aggregation [22], upregulation of the expression of CD11b, or shedding of CD62L from the cell surface [13].

Materials and Methods

Monoclonal Antibodies

Anti-CD9 mAb (MM2/57, IgG2b) and anti-CD53 mAb (MEM-53, IgG1) were purchased from Serotec (Oxon, UK). Anti-CD37 mAb (HD28, IgG2b), anti-CD63 mAb (H5C6, IgG1) and anti-CD81 mAb (5A6, IgG1) were obtained as a result of our participation in the 5th International Workshop on Leukocyte Differentiation Antigens [23]. Irrelevant IgG1 control antibody (MOPC 21, IgG1) was purchased from Sigma Chemical Co. (St. Louis, Mo., USA). R-Phycoerythrin (PE)-conjugated mAbs, anti-CD11b mAb (Leu-15, IgG2a) and anti-CD62L mAb (Leu-8, IgG2a), or PE-conjugated irrelevant IgG2a control antibody were purchased from Becton Dickinson (Mountain View, Calif., USA).

Isolation of Human Eosinophils

Eosinophils were purified from peripheral blood of allergic donors using Percoll (Pharmacia, Uppsala, Sweden) density gradient centrifugation followed by negative selection with anti-CD16 mAb (clone 3G8, IgG1, Medarex, West Lebanon, N.H., USA) along with immunomagnetic beads coated with goat anti-mouse IgG (Dynabeads M450, Dynal, Oslo, Norway) as previously described [24]. The purity and viability of eosinophils were determined by light-microscopic examination of cytocentrifugation preparations (Shandon, Pittsburgh, Pa., USA) stained by Diff-Quik (American Scientific Products, McGraw Park, Ill., USA) and by erythrocin B dye exclusion (Sigma). Both were consistently greater than 96 and 99%, respectively (n = 6).

Flow-Cytometric Analysis of Cell Surface TM4SF Expression

Expression of TM4SF molecules on eosinophils was examined using indirect immunofluorescence and flow cytometry as previously described [25]. Briefly, freshly isolated eosinophils were washed twice with Dulbecco's PBS containing 0.1% bovine serum albumin (Sigma, PBS-BSA), and incubated (30 min, 4°C in PBS-BSA) with 4 mg/ml human IgG (Sigma) and saturating concentrations of mAb or an equivalent concentration of irrelevant IgG1 control mAb. Cells were washed 3 times and then incubated (30 min, 4°C in PBS-BSA) with 1:50 dilutions of PE-conjugated F(ab')2 goat anti-mouse IgG antibody (Tago, Burlingame, Calif., USA). After fixation with 1% paraformaldehyde (Sigma) in PBS, at least 8,000 cells were evaluated

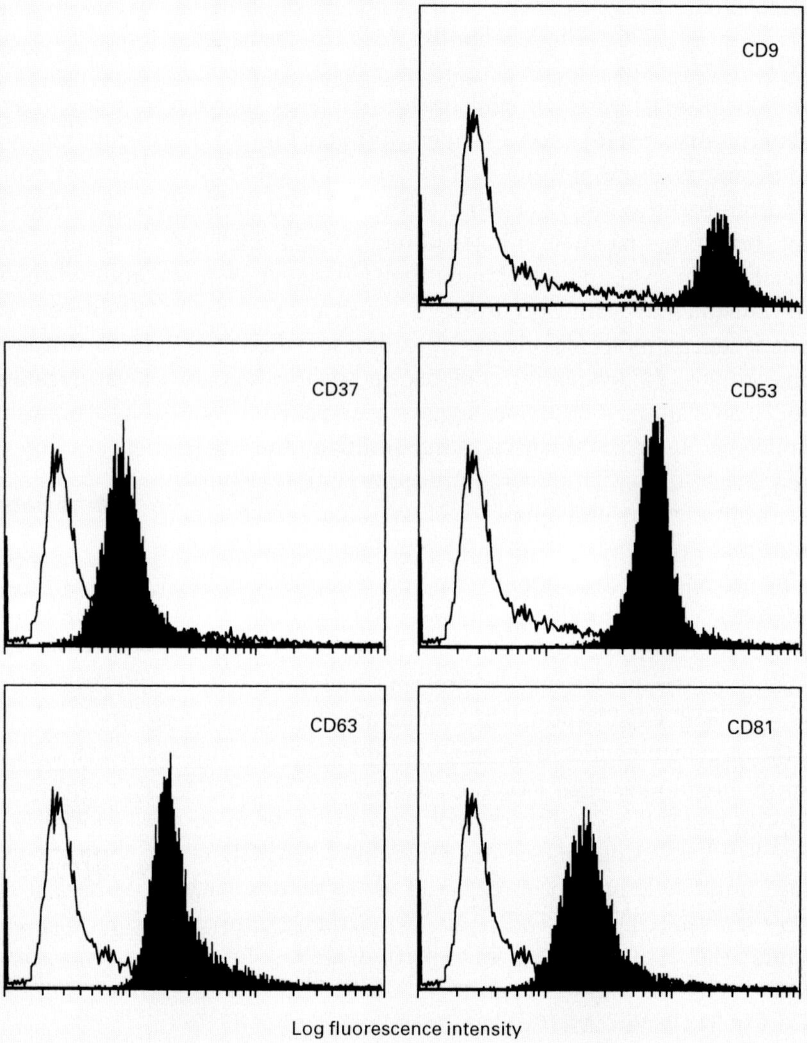

Fig. 1. Expression of TM4SF molecules on freshly isolated human eosinophils. The shaded histogram shows the expression of each TM4SF molecule. Data are from one experiment representative of four experiments with different donors; the solid line represents labeling with an irrelevant IgG1 antibody.

using an EPICS Profile flow cytometer (Coulter, Hialeah, Fla., USA).

Eosinophil Culture

Eosinophils were cultured as previously described [26]. In brief, eosinophils were suspended in RPMI 1640 medium (Gibco BRL, Grand Island, N.Y., USA) supplemented with 10% fetal bovine serum (High Clone Laboratories, Logan, Utah, USA), 100 U/ml penicillin G, 100 mg/ml streptomycin, and 0.25 mg/ml amphotericin B (Gibco BRL) at a density of 5×10^5/ml. Cells were cultured for up to 24 h in the presence of 10^{-7} *M* platelet-activating factor (PAF, Sigma), 10 μg/ml anti-TM4SF mAb or irrelevant control IgG1 mAb at 37 °C in a humidified atmosphere containing 95% air and 5% CO_2 in 24-well sterile flat-bottom plates (Costar, Cambridge, Mass., USA). Recovery and viability always exceeded 90 and 81%, respectively.

Flow-Cytometric Analysis of Homotypic Aggregation of Eosinophils

Flow-cytometric analysis for the homotypic aggregation of eosinophils was performed by using the dot plot histogram of forward scatter and side scatter as previously described [27]. The percentage of cells excluded from the original single cell region was then calculated and considered to be aggregated cells. This analysis was done 3–4 times with different donors.

Flow-Cytometric Analysis of Cell Surface CD11b or CD62L Expression

Expression of CD11b or CD62L on eosinophils was examined using direct immunofluorescence and flow cytometry as previously described [28]. Briefly, harvested eosinophils were washed with PBS-BSA and incubated (30 min, 4 °C in PBS-BSA) with 4 mg/ml human IgG and saturating concentrations of PE-conjugated anti-CD11b,

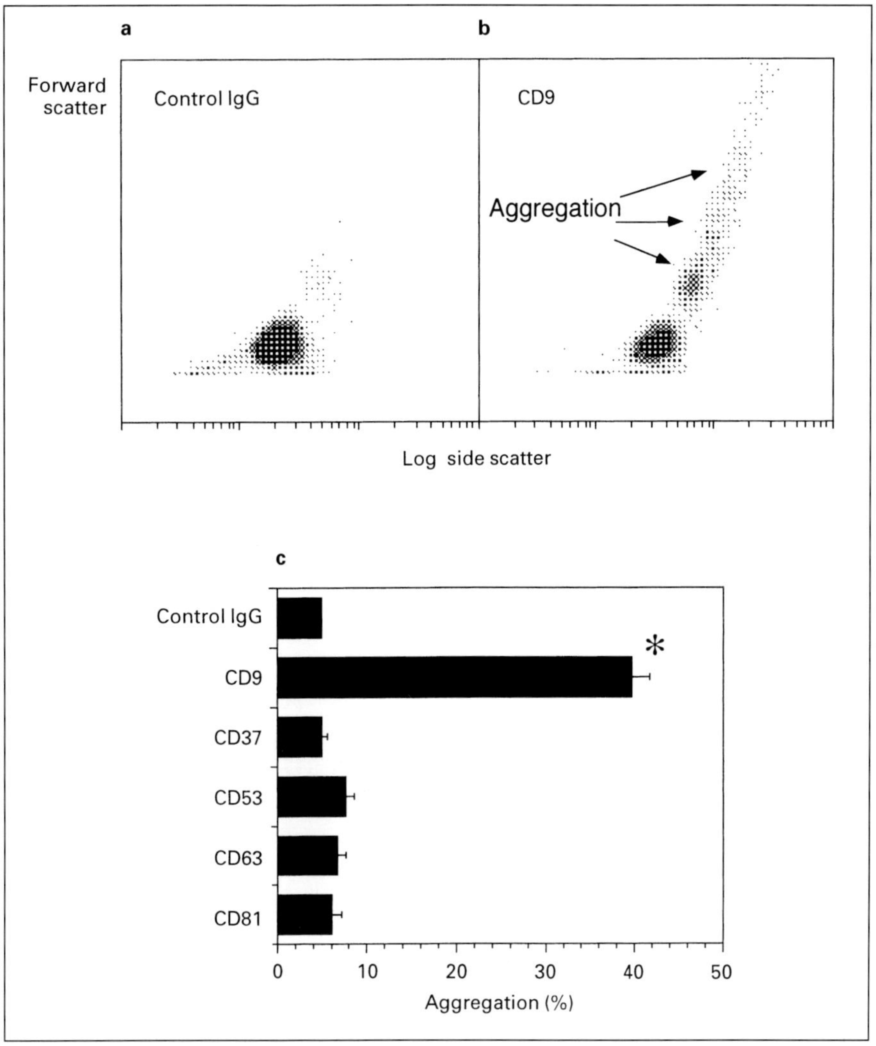

Fig. 2. Homotypic aggregation of eosinophils after cross-linking of TM4SF molecules on eosinophils. **a**, **b** Homotypic aggregation of eosinophils was assessed by using flow cytometry. **a** Dot plot with forward scatter and side scatter. Note that the distribution of control mAb-treated eosinophil formed a single population of single cells. **b** After incubation with anti-CD9 mAb, the pattern of eosinophil light scatter now consists of both single cells and multiple cell aggregates. The percentage of the cells outside of the single cell population was then determined and considered to be aggregated cells. **c** Among all mAbs against TM4SF molecules, only anti-CD9 mAb showed significant eosinophil homotypic aggregation after 30 min of culture. * $p < 0.001$ (n = 3–4).

anti-CD62L mAb or an equivalent concentration of PE-conjugated irrelevant IgG2a control mAb. After subsequent washing, fixation and flow-cytometric analysis were performed.

Statistical Analysis

Data are presented as the mean ± SEM. Statistical significance was determined by Student's t test or paired t test and considered significant for $p < 0.05$.

Results

Expression of TM4SF Molecules on Eosinophils

As shown in figure 1, freshly isolated peripheral blood eosinophils constitutively expressed CD9, CD37, CD53, CD63 and CD81. The flow-cytometric histograms of fresh eosinophils from all 4 donors consistently showed a unimodal peak of staining with each of these anti-TM4SF mAbs, and were statistically different when compared to the irrelevant IgG1 control antibody. Fresh eosinophils constitutively express CD9, CD37, CD53, CD63 and CD81 [irrelevant IgG1 control mean fluorescent intensity (MFI): 2.9 ± 0.3; CD9 MFI: 475.3 ± 17.3*; CD37 MFI: 23.9 ± 2.7*; CD53 MFI: 47.7 ± 10.9*; CD63 MFI: 23.6 ± 2.6*; CD81 MFI: 13.6 ± 3.3*; * $p < 0.05$; n = 4]. Their MFI did not change after the incubation of eosinophils with 10^{-7} *M* PAF for 30 min (data not shown).

Eosinophil Homotypic Aggregation after Cross-Linking of TM4SF

Incubation for 30 min with anti-CD9 mAb, but not with anti-CD37, CD53, CD63 or CD81 mAb, induced significant eosinophil homotypic aggregation (fig. 2).

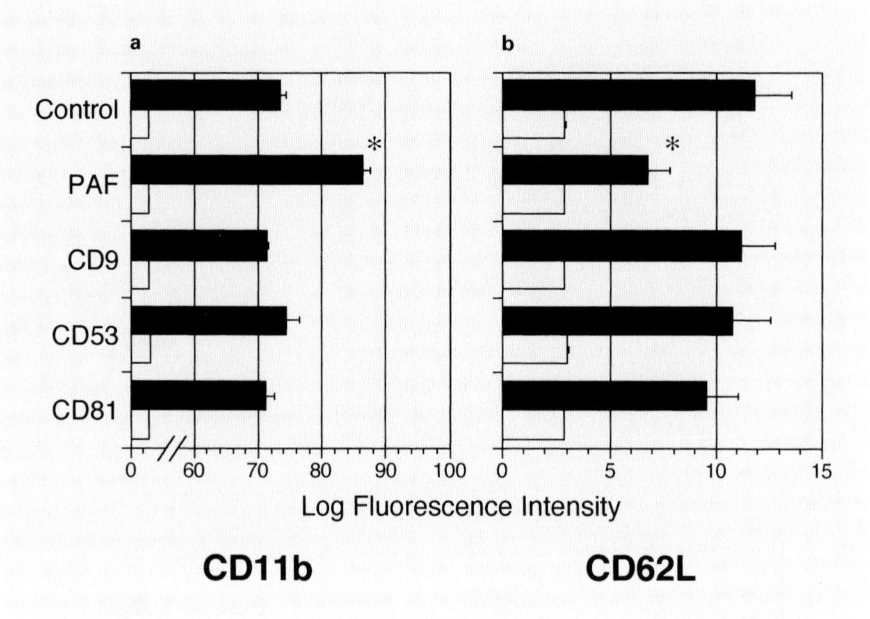

Fig. 3. Effect of 30 min incubation with anti-TM4SF mAbs on eosinophil expression of CD11b (**a**) and CD62L (**b**). □ = MFI of irrelevant IgG2a control; ■ = MFI of CD11b (**a**) or CD62L (**b**). 10^{-7} *M* PAF, used as a positive control, significantly enhanced CD11b expression and significantly reduced CD62L expression. * $p < 0.05$ (n = 3–4). None of the anti-TM4SF mAbs altered CD11b or CD62L on eosinophils. In all experiments, MFI with irrelevant IgG2a remained unchanged.

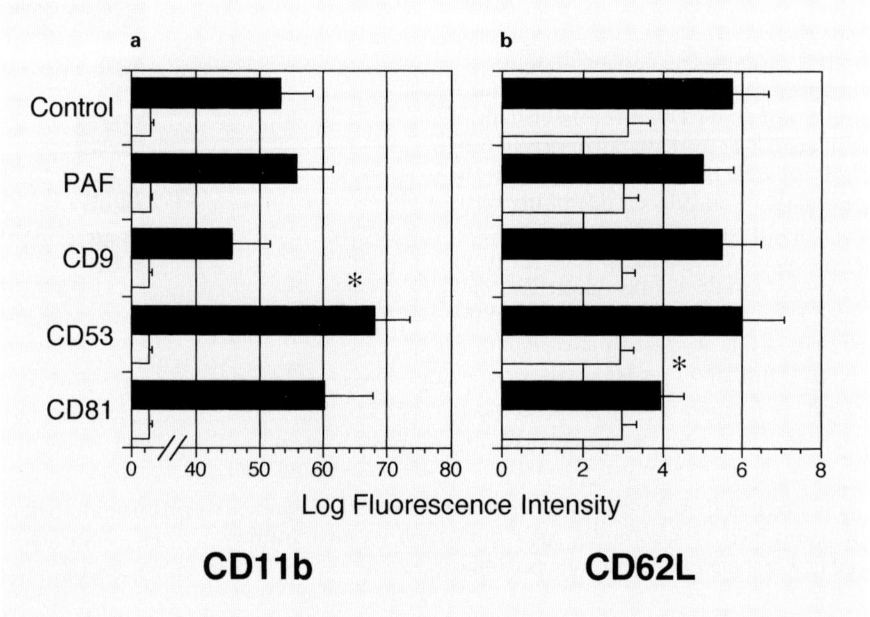

Fig. 4. Effect of 24 h incubation with anti-TM4SF mAbs on eosinophil expression of CD11b (**a**) and CD62L (**b**). □ = MFI of irrelevant IgG2a control; ■ MFI of CD11b (**a**) or CD62L (**b**). After 24 h of culture with mAbs against CD53, the expression of CD11b on eosinophils was significantly enhanced (**a**). In addition, the expression of CD62L was significantly reduced when eosinophils were cultured with anti-CD81 mAb (**b**). * $p < 0.05$ (n = 3–4). In all experiments, MFI with irrelevant IgG2a was not changed.

Treatment of eosinophils with PAF for 30 min also failed to induce eosinophil homotypic aggregation (data not shown).

Effect of PAF or TM4SF Cross-Linking on Eosinophil Expression of CD11b and CD62L

After incubation with 10^{-7} *M* for 30 min, CD11b expression on eosinophil was significantly enhanced whereas the expression of CD62L was reduced as expected (fig. 3). In contrast, incubation with anti-TM4SF mAb for 30 min did not alter the expression of either CD11b or CD62L on eosinophils. However, the expression of CD11b was significantly enhanced after 24 h of incubation with mAbs against CD53 when compared with the eosinophils cultured with irrelevant IgG1 control (fig. 4a). In addition, the expression of CD62L was significantly reduced with anti-CD81 mAbs (fig. 4b).

Discussion

Most members of the TM4SF are implicated in the activation of various types of cells, including pre-B cells, platelets and T cells. However, little is known about their role in granulocyte function. In the present study, we have demonstrated that freshly isolated eosinophils express several members of the TM4SF including CD9, CD37, CD53, CD63 and CD81, confirming a previous report [23].

Cross-linking of eosinophil surface CD9 induced significant homotypic aggregation of eosinophils, while mAb to other TM4SF molecules tested had no effect. Surprisingly, CD81, expressed on eosinophils but not on neutrophils [23] and the molecule with the highest homology to CD9, failed to induce homotypic aggregation upon cross-linking by mAb, especially since CD81 cross-linking has been reported to induce homotypic aggregation of B cells [29].

Kim et al. [20] showed that cross-linking of eosinophil surface CD9 with immobilized or soluble mAb had a different effect on eosinophils; the former induced degranulation while the latter induced secretion of GM-CSF. They also reported that this effect was found in some but not all mAbs against CD9. These data strongly suggest that CD9 might be functionally or physically associated with eosinophil β_1 or β_2 integrins. The specific mechanisms of eosinophil homotypic aggregation after ligation of CD9 are still unknown and require further study.

Among the TM4SF members tested, culture of eosinophils with mAb against CD53 for 24 h induced significant upregulation of CD11b expression. As eosinophil binding via CD11b is crucial for eosinophil degranulation [10], enhanced CD11b expression may result in functional alterations of eosinophils. On the other hand, cross-linking of eosinophil surface CD81 for 24 h induced significant shedding of CD62L.

In terms of kinetics, upon cross-linking of TM4SF molecules on eosinophils, CD11b upregulation or CD62L shedding consistent with eosinophil activation was observed by 24 h but not 30 min in vitro. It has been reported that degranulation of eosinophils occurs 4 h after cross-linking of eosinophil surface CD9 with immobilized mAb [20]. A possible explanation for the difference in the time kinetics of the effect of anti-TM4SF mAb treatment might be differences in TM4SF molecule cross-linking. Kim et al. used coated tissue culture plates, whereas we used mAbs without any secondary antibody cross-linking.

In the present study, we demonstrated that human eosinophils express several TM4SF molecules including CD9, CD37, CD53, CD63 and CD81. Among these molecules, mAb to CD9, CD53 and CD81 are capable of activating different functions of eosinophils. These data suggest that the mechanisms of homotypic aggregation, CD11b upregulation and CD62L shedding are distinct, and it is possible that the associated molecule for TM4SF molecules on eosinophils is not the same. The specific molecules physically and functionally associated with TM4SF molecules on eosinophils, or the specific mAbs that are capable of regulating eosinophil function must now be identified in further studies. Once clarified, the molecules may prove to be potent targets for the regulation of allergic inflammation.

Acknowledgment

This work was supported in part by grant HL49545 from the National Institutes of Health, a Developing Investigator Award (to B.S.B.) from the Burroughs Wellcome Fund, and the Japan-North America Medical Exchange Foundation (to K.M.).

References

1 Gleich GJ: The eosinophil and bronchial asthma: Current understanding. J Allergy Clin Immunol 1990;85:422–436.
2 Silberstein DS, David JR: The regulation of human eosinophil function by cytokines. Immunol Today 1987;8:380–385.
3 Hirai K, Miyamasu M, Takaishi T, Morita Y: Regulation of the function of eosinophils and basophils. Crit Rev Immunol 1997;17:325–352.
4 Springer TA: Adhesion receptors of the immune system. Nature 1990;346:425–434.
5 Weber C, Katayama J, Springer TA: Differential regulation of β1 and β2 integrin avidity by chemoattractants in eosinophils. Proc Natl Acad Sci USA 1996;93:10939–10944.
6 Schleimer RP, Sterbinsky SA, Kaiser J, Bickel CA, Klunk DA, Tomioka K, Newman W, Luscinskas FW, Gimbrone MA Jr, McIntyre BW, Bochner BS: Interleukin-4 induces adherence of human eosinophils and basophils but not neutrophils to endothelium: Association with expression of VCAM-1. J Immunol 1992;148:1086–1092.
7 Nagata M, Sedgwick JB, Bates ME, Kita H, Busse WW: Eosinophil adhesion to vascular cell adhesion molecule-1 activates superoxide anion generation. J Immunol 1995;155:2194–2202.
8 Anwar ARF, Moqbel R, Walsh GM, Kay AB, Wardlaw AJ: Adhesion to fibronectin prolongs eosinophil survival. J Exp Med 1993;177:839–843.
9 Anwar ARE, Walsh GM, Cromwell O, Kay AB, Wardlaw AJ: Adhesion to fibronectin primes eosinophil via α4/β1 (VLA-4). Immunology 1994;82:222–228.

10 Horie S, Kita H: CD11b/CD18 (Mac-1) is required for degranulation of human eosinophils induced by human recombinant granulocyte-macrophage colony-stimulating factor and platelet-activating factor. J Immunol 1994;152: 5457–5467.
11 Hynes RO: Integrins: Versatility, modulation, and signaling in cell adhesion. Cell 1992;69: 11–25.
12 Matsumoto K, Sterbinsky SA, Bickel CA, Zhou DFH, Kovach NL, Bochner BS: Regulation of α4 integrin-mediated adhesion of human eosinophils to fibronectin and vascular cell adhesion molecule-1. J Allergy Clin Immunol 1997; 99:648–656.
13 Matsumoto K, Bochner BS, Wakiguchi H, Kurashige T: Altered expression of CD11b and CD62L after cross-linking of CD45 isoforms on human eosinophils. Int Arch Allergy Immunol 1998;117:S34–39.
14 Wright MD, Tomlinson MG: The ins and outs of the transmembrane 4 superfamily. Immunol Today 1994;15:588–594.
15 Rubinstein E, Le NF, Lagaudriere GC, Billard M, Conjeaud H, Boucheix C: CD9, CD63, CD81, and CD82 are components of a surface tetraspan network connected to HLA-DR and VLA integrins. Eur J Immunol 1996;26:2657–2665.
16 Rubinstein E, Le NF, Billard M, Prenant M, Boucheix C: CD9 antigen is an accessory subunit of the VLA integrin complexes. Eur J Immunol 1994;24:3005–3013.
17 Mannion BA, Berditchevski F, Kraeft SK, Chen LB, Hemler ME: Transmembrane-4 superfamily proteins CD81 (TAPA-1), CD82, CD63, and CD53 specifically associated with integrin α4β1 (CD49d/CD29). J Immunol 1996;157:2039–2047.
18 Skubitz KM, Campbell KD, Iida J, Skubitz AP: CD63 associates with tyrosine kinase activity and CD11/CD18, and transmits an activation signal in neutrophils. J Immunol 1996;157: 3617–3626.
19 Maecker HT, Todd SC, Levy S: The tetraspanin superfamily: Molecular facilitators. FASEB J 1997;11:428–442.
20 Kim JT, Gleich GJ, Kita H: Roles of CD9 molecules in survival and activation of human eosinophils. J Immunol 1997;159:926–933.
21 Masellis SA, Shaw AR: CD9-regulated adhesion. Anti-CD9 monoclonal antibody induces pre-B cell adhesion to bone marrow fibroblasts through de novo recognition of fibronectin. J Immunol 1994;152:2768–2777.
22 Masellis SA, Jensen GS, Seehafer JG, Slupsky JR, Shaw AR: Anti-CD9 monoclonal antibodies induce homotypic adhesion of pre-B cell lines by a novel mechanism. J Immunol 1990; 144:1607–1613.
23 Ebisawa M, Schleimer RP, Bickel CA, Bochner BS: Phenotyping of purified human peripheral blood eosinophils using the blind panel mAb; in Schlossman S, Boumsell L, Gilks W, Harlan J, Kishimoto T, Morimoto C, Ritz J, Shaw S, Silverstein R, Springer T, Tedder T, Todd R (eds): Leukocyte Typing V: White Cell Differentiation Antigens. New York, Oxford University Press, 1995, pp 1036–1038.
24 Hansel TT, Pound JD, Pilling D, Kitas GD, Salmon M, Gentle TA, Lee SS, Thompson RA: Purification of human eosinophils by negative selection using immunomagnetic beads. J Immunol Methods 1989;122:97–103.
25 Bochner BS, McKelvey AA, Schleimer RP, Hildreth JEK, MacGlashan DW Jr: Flow cytometric methods for analysis of human basophil surface antigens and viability. J Immunol Methods 1989;125:265–271.
26 Matsumoto K, Schleimer RP, Saito H, Iikura Y, Bochner BS: Induction of apoptosis in human eosinophils by anti-Fas antibody treatment in vitro. Blood 1995;86:1437–1443.
27 Peter MJ, Heyderman RS, Hatch DJ, Klein NJ: Investigation of platelet-neutrophil interactions in whole blood by flow cytometry. J Immunol Methods 1997;209:125–135.
28 Bochner BS, Sterbinsky SA: Altered surface expression of CD11 and Leu 8 during human basophil degranulation. J Immunol 1991;146: 2367–2373.
29 Takahashi S, Doss C, Levy S, Levy R: TAPA-1, the target of an antiproliferative antibody, is associated on the cell surface with the Leu-13 antigen. J Immunol 1990;145:2207–2213.

International Archives of
Allergy and
Immunology

Int Arch Allergy Immunol 1999;120(suppl 1):45–47

CCR3 mRNA Expression in Bronchial Epithelial Cells and Various Cells in Allergic Inflammation

Hajime Oyamada[a] Yumiko Kamada[a] Tomoe Kuwasaki[a]
Yoshiyuki Yamada[b] Yoshimi Kobayashi[b] Chang-Hao Cui[b] Kohei Honda[b]
Hiroyuki Kayaba[b] Norihiro Saito[b] Junichi Chihara[b]

[a]Division of Central Laboratory, Akita University Hospital, and [b]Department of Clinical and Laboratory Medicine, Akita University School of Medicine, Akita, Japan

Key Words

CCR3 · Eotaxin · RT-PCR · Allergic inflammation · Bronchial epithelium · Eosinophils

Abstract

Background: RANTES and eotaxin are important chemokines involved in the activation and migration of eosinophils and are considered to play a major role in allergic inflammation. ***Methods:*** In this study, we used RT-PCR to investigate the kinds of cells that express mRNA for CCR3, a common receptor of these chemokines, and eotaxin, a ligand for CCR3. ***Results:*** CCR3 mRNA was expressed in eosinophils, peripheral mononuclear cells, an eosinophilic cell line (EoL-1), a bronchial epithelial cell line ($NCI\text{-}H_{292}$), human endothelial cells and nasal washings from patients with allergic rhinitis. ***Conclusion:*** These results suggest that the CCR3-eotaxin system plays an important role in generating inflammation, since these substances are expressed not only in cells implicated in activation or migration of eosinophils but also in various other cells involved in allergic inflammation.

Introduction

Infiltration of diverse inflammatory cells is observed at allergic inflammation sites such as those in asthma. In particular, eosinophils are the main constituent of the infiltrates, and are considered to play an important role in allergic inflammation.

Since RANTES and eotaxin were recently discovered to be chemokines that participate in selective migration and activation of eosinophils, the kinetics of these substances have been studied [1–3].

In this study, we used RT-PCR to investigate the type of cells expressing mRNA for CCR3, a common receptor for RANTES and eotaxin. mRNA expression of eotaxin, a ligand for CCR3, was also examined. Moreover, we examined whether a reaction system mediated by CCR3 is present at allergic inflammation sites using nasal washings from patients with allergic rhinitis.

Material and Methods

Cells and Cell Lines

Eosinophils were isolated from heparinized peripheral venous blood obtained from patients with hypereosinophilic syndrome by a modified CD16-negative depletion method as previously described [4]. Peripheral mononuclear cells (PMC) were isolated from heparinized peripheral venous blood obtained from normal controls by

KARGER

Fax + 41 61 306 12 34
E-Mail karger@karger.ch
www.karger.com

1018–2438/99/1205–0045$17.50/0

Accessible online at:
http://BioMedNet.com/karger

Dr. Junichi Chihara
Department of Clinical and Laboratory Medicine
Akita University School of Medicine
Hondo Akita 010-8543 (Japan)
Tel. +81 18 834 1111, Fax +81 18 836 2624

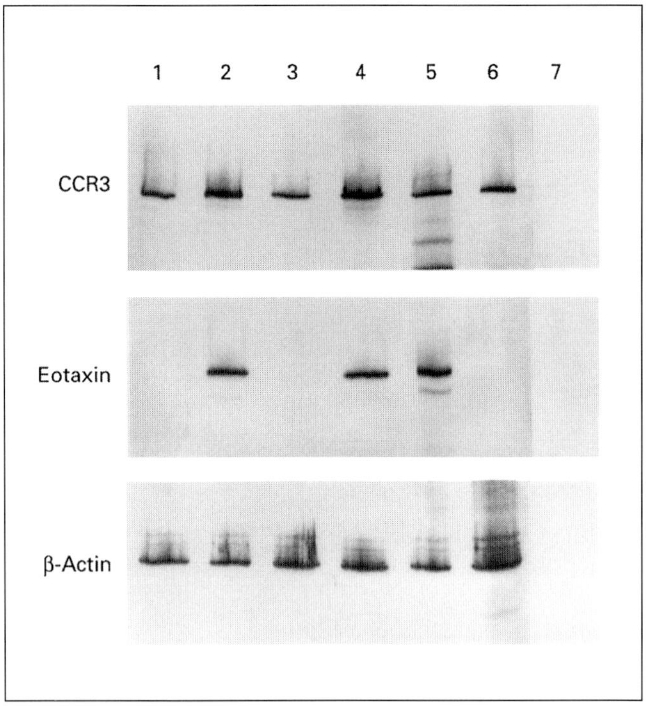

Fig. 1. RT-PCR analysis of CCR3 and eotaxin mRNA expression in various cells/cell lines. Lane 1: purified eosinophils; lane 2: PMCs; lane 3: EoL-1; lane 4: ECs; lane 5: bronchial epithelial cell line; lane 6: CCR3 transfectant cells; lane 7: negative control (H_2O). The amplified products were separated on 12.5% polyacrylamide gel stained with silver staining.

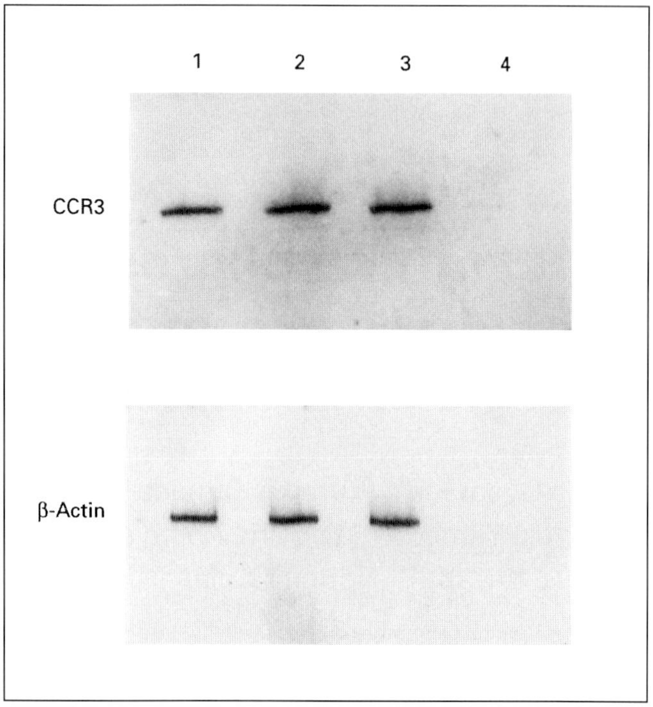

Fig. 2. RT-PCR analysis of CCR3 mRNA expression in nasal washings of patients with allergic rhinitis and normal controls. Lanes 1 and 2: normal controls; lane 3: patients with allergic rhinitis; lane 4: negative control (H_2O). The amplified products were separated on 12.5% polyacrylamide gel stained with silver staining.

Ficoll-Paque gradient centrifugation (specific gravity 1.077 g/ml; Pharmacia Biotech, Uppsala, Sweden). CCR3 transfectants were K562 cells expressing CCR3 (supplied by Dr. Osamu Yoshie, Shionogi Institute for Medical Science, Osaka, Japan). EoL-1 and NCI-H_{292} are cell lines derived from human eosinophilic leukemia cells [5] and human bronchial epithelial cells [6] (American Type Culture Collection, Rockville, Md., USA), respectively. Human endothelial cells (ECS) were obtained from umbilical cord vein by collagenase and transformed with SV-40 [7]. For nasal washings, both nasal cavities of patients with allergic rhinitis and normal subjects were slowly washed with 5 ml of physiological saline 10 times each. After the washings were mixed and centrifuged at 1,500 rpm, the sediments were used for examination.

RT-PCR Analysis

Polyadenylated RNA was extracted (QuickPrep mRNA Purification Kit, Pharmacia Biotech) and reverse-transcribed using a SuperScript II Preamplification System (Gibco-BRL, Gaithersburg, Md., USA). One microliter of cDNA synthesis reaction was used as a template for PCR amplification with AmpliTaq DNA polymerase (Perkin-Elmer, Foster City, Calif., USA). The CCR3 primers were 5′-TCCTTCTCTCTTCCTATCAATC-3′ and 5′-GGCAATTTTCTGCATCTG-3′ [8]. The eotaxin primers were 5′-CCCAACCACCTGCTGCTTTAACCTG-3′ and 5′-TGGCTTTGGAGTTGGAGATTTTGG-3′ [9]. The β-actin primers were purchased from Clontech (Palo Alto, Calif., USA). The PCR cycle consisted of 45 s denaturation at 94 °C, 45 s annealing at 55 °C (for CCR3) or 57 °C (for eotaxin) and 1 min extension at 72 °C for 35 cycles.

Results

Analysis of CCR3 mRNA expression in a variety of cells using RT-PCR revealed that CCR3 mRNA was expressed in purified eosinophils, PMCs, an eosinophilic cell line (EoL-1), a bronchial epithelial cell line (NCI-H_{292}), and ECs. When mRNA expression of eotaxin, which is a ligand for CCR3, was investigated in the same cells, eotaxin mRNA was expressed in PMCs, a bronchial epithelial cell line and ECs (fig. 1).

To examine the involvement of CCR3 at the actual sites of allergic inflammation, mRNA expressions of CCR3 in cells from nasal washings of patients with allergic rhinitis were studied. CCR3 mRNA was expressed in nasal washings from both normal subjects and patients (fig. 2).

Discussion

CCR3 was initially cloned from eosinophils [10], and the expression in basophils was reported thereafter [11]. This study using RT-PCR demonstrates that, in addition to these cells, PMCs, an eosinophilic cell line, a bronchial epithelial cell line and ECs also expressed CCR3.

Bonecchi et al. [12] reported that CCR3 was present in peripheral mononuclear cells, consistent with our results. A recent study by Tiffany et al. [13] demonstrated that another eosinophilic cell line (HL-60) expressed CCR3 when the cells were differentiated and matured using butyric acid, as opposed to our results using a nonstimulated eosinophilic cell line. This discrepancy may be due to differences in the properties of these cell lines or those in the sensitivity for detection between Northern blot analysis used by Tiffany et al. [13] and RT-PCR used by us.

Few studies have described CCR3 expression on epithelial cells such as NCI-H_{292} and ECs. CCR3 protein expression on these cells was confirmed by flow cytometry and immunohistochemistry using anti-CCR3 monoclonal antibodies (data not shown). The mRNA expression of eotaxin, a specific ligand for CCR3, was confirmed in PMCs, a bronchial epithelial cell line, and ECs.

Ying et al. [14] documented that eotaxin was expressed in epithelial cells, endothelial cells, macrophages, T cells and mast cells in detailed experiments using bronchial biopsy samples from asthmatic patients. In addition to these cells, eotaxin expression was also noted in eosinophils in similar experiments by Mattoli et al. [15].

However, in this study, we could not confirm eotaxin expression in highly purified eosinophils. As material from allergic inflammation sites, nasal washings from patients with allergic rhinitis and normal subjects were tested for CCR3 mRNA. CCR3 was expressed in nasal washings from both groups of subjects.

Our data suggest that the CCR3-eotaxin reaction system plays an important role in generating inflammation, since these substances are expressed not only in cells implicated in the activation or migration of eosinophils but also in various other cells involved in allergic inflammation.

Besides the expression of mRNA, we also observed the surface expression of CCR3 using monoclonal antibody (manuscript in preparation). The details of CCR3 expression require further investigation by Western or Northern blotting.

References

1 Kakazu T, Chihara J, Saito A, Nakajima S: Effect of RANTES on eosinophilic adhesion to plates coated with recombinant soluble intercellular adhesion molecule-1 and expression of β_2-integrin adhesion molecules on eosinophils. Int Arch Allergy Immunol 1995;108(suppl 1): 9–11.

2 Yamada H, Izutani R, Chihara J, Yudate T, Matsukura M, Tezuka T: RANTES mRNA expression in skin and colon of patients with atopic dermatitis. Int Arch Allergy Immunol 1996;111(suppl 1):19–21.

3 Chihara J, Oyamada H, Yamada H, Tsuda A, Kamada Y, Urayama O: Expression of mRNA for RANTES in human eosinophils. Int Arch Allergy Immunol 1997;114(suppl 1):33–35.

4 Chihara J, Kurachi D, Yamada H, Wada T, Yasukawa A, Nakajima S: A comparative study of isolation of eosinophils by different procedures of CD16 negative depletion. Allergy 1995;50:11–14.

5 Chihara J, Kurachi Dai, Yamamoto T, Higashimoto I, Kakazu T, Nakajima S: Induction of β2 integrin expression on an eosinophilic cell line (EoL-1) by the supernatant of mononuclear cells stimulated with specific allergen from asthmatic patients. Immunol Lett 1994; 42:25–29.

6 Chihara J, Urayama O, Tsuda A, Kakazu T, Hiagasimoto I, Yamada H: Eosinophil cationic protein induces insulin-like growth factor I receptor expression on bronchial epithelial cells. Int Arch Allergy Immunol 1996;111(suppl 1): 43–45.

7 Chihara J, Maruyama I, Yasuba H, Yasukawa A, Yamamoto T, Kurachi D, Mouri T, Seguchi M, Nakajima S: Possible induction of intercellular adhesion molecule-1 (ICAM-1) expression on endothelial cells by platelet-activating factor (PAF). J Lipid Mediat 1992;5:159–162.

8 He J, Chen Y, Farzan M, Choe H, Ohagen A, Gartner S, Busciglio J, Yang X, Hofmann W, Mackay CR, Sodroski J, Gabuzda D: CCR3 and CCR5 are co-receptor for HIV-1 infection of microglia. Nature 1997;385:645–649.

9 Bartels J, Schluter C, Richter E, Noso N, Kulke R, Christophers E, Schröder JM: Human dermal fibroblasts express eotaxin: Molecular mRNA expression, and identification of eotaxin sequence variants. Biochem Biophys Res Commun 1996;225:1045–1051.

10 Daugherty BL, Siciliano SJ, DeMartino JA, Malkowitz L, Sirotina A, Springer MS: Cloning, expression, and characterization of the human eosinophil eotaxin receptor. J Exp Med 1996;183:2349–2354.

11 Yamada H, Hirai K, Miyamasu M, Iikura M, Misaki Y, Shoji S, Takahasi T, Kasahara T, Morita Y, Ito K: Eotaxin is a potent chemotaxin for human basophils. Biochem Biophys Res Commun 1997;236:365–368.

12 Bonecchi R, Bianchi G, Bordignon PP, D'Ambrosio D, Lang R, Borsatti A, Sozzani S, Allavena P, Gray PA, Mantovani A, Sinigaglia F: Differential expression of chemokine receptors and chemotactic responsiveness of type 1 T helper cells (Th1s) and Th2s. J Exp Med 1998; 187:129–134.

13 Tiffany HL, Alkhatib G, Combadiere C, Berger EA, Murphy PM: CC chemokine receptor 1 and 3 are differentially regulated by IL-5 during maturation of eosinophilic HL-60 cells. J Immunol 1998;160:1385–1392.

14 Ying S, Robinson DS, Meng Q, Rottman J, Kennedy R, Ringler DJ, Mackay CR, Daugherty BL, Springer MS, Durham SR, Williams TJ, Kay AB: Enhanced expression of eotaxin and CCR3 mRNA and protein in atopic asthma. Association with airway hyperresponsiveness and predominant co-localization of eotaxin mRNA to bronchial epithelial and endothelial cells. Eur J Immunol 1997;27:3507–3516.

15 Mattoli S, Stacey MA, Sun G, Bellini A, Marini M: Eotaxin expression and eosinophilic inflammation in asthma. Biochem Biophys Res Commun 1997;236:299–301.

International Archives of
Allergy and Immunology

Int Arch Allergy Immunol 1999;120(suppl 1):48–50

Effect of Eotaxin on the Generation of Reactive Oxygen Species from Eosinophil Cell Line, YY-1

Kohei Honda[a] Yoshiyuki Yamada[a] Chang-Hao Cui[a] Norihoro Saito[a]
Hiroyuki Kayaba[a] Yoshimi Kobayashi[a] Hajime Oyamada[b]
Yumiko Kamada[b] Tomoe Kuwasaki[b] Susumu Tsurufuji[c] Junichi Chihara[a]

[a]Department of Clinical and Laboratory Medicine, Akita University School of Medicine, Hondo, Akita,
[b]Division of Central Laboratory, Akita University Hospital, Akita, and [c]Cytosignal Institute, Tokyo, Japan

Key Words
Luminol-dependent chemiluminescence · Chemokines · Eosinophils · Reactive oxygen species · Eotaxin · YY-1

Abstract
Background: The CC chemokine eotaxin is a selective chemoattractant for eosinophils. Eosinophils have been considered to be the major effector cells in allergic inflammation, since not only eosinophil-specific granule proteins but also reactive oxygen species (ROS) from eosinophils may cause the damage to the cells or tissue of the mucosal epithelium. In this study, we examined the effect of eotaxin on ROS from an eosinophil cell line, YY-1. ***Methods:*** ROS in luminol-dependent reaction were examined. Calcium ionophore A23187 were added to the mixture of YY-1 cells with luminol, and then ROS were determined. ***Results:*** Eotaxin primed the production of ROS from YY-1 cells. ROS from untreated YY-1 cells evoked with calcium ionophore A23187 in luminol-dependent chemiluminescence gave a maximal value of 1,928 ± 223 intensity counts (IC; mean ± SE, n = 4) and an integral value of 17.04 ± 1.51 IC ($\times 10^{-4}$), while eosinophils that were treated with eotaxin gave a maximal value of 2,264 ± 86 IC (10 n*M*), 2,691 ± 124 IC (100 n*M*) and an integral value of 21.22 ± 0.67 IC ($\times 10^{-4}$; 10 n*M*), 26.20 ± 1.41 IC ($\times 10^{-4}$; 100 n*M*). ***Conclusion:*** Eotaxin might play important roles in the pathogenesis of allergic inflammation through eosinophil activation by priming of eosinophil oxidative metabolism as well as involvement in selective eosinophil chemotaxis.

Introduction

It is well known that increased numbers of eosinophils or deposition of eosinophil-specific granules are observed in the inflamed tissues in allergic inflammation, such as bronchial asthma. Eosinophils are considered to be major inflammatory cells in allergic reaction [1], since eosinophil-specific granule proteins damage the mucosal epithelium [2].

Recently, a new family of chemotactic cytokines, chemokines, have been identified [3]. The chemokines, secreted 8- to 10-kD proteins, activate and attract leukocytes to inflammatory foci through binding to specific G protein-coupled seven transmembrane-spanning cell surface receptors [4]. The chemokine are mainly divided into the two subfamilies, CC chemokine and CXC chemokine

KARGER
Fax +41 61 306 12 34
E-Mail karger@karger.ch
www.karger.com

1018–2438/99/1205–0048$17.50/0

Accessible online at:
http://BioMedNet.com/karger

Dr. Junichi Chihara
Department of Clinical and Laboratory Medicine
Akita University School of Medicine
Hondo, Akita 010-8543 (Japan)
Tel. +81 18 834 1111, Fax +81 18 836 2624

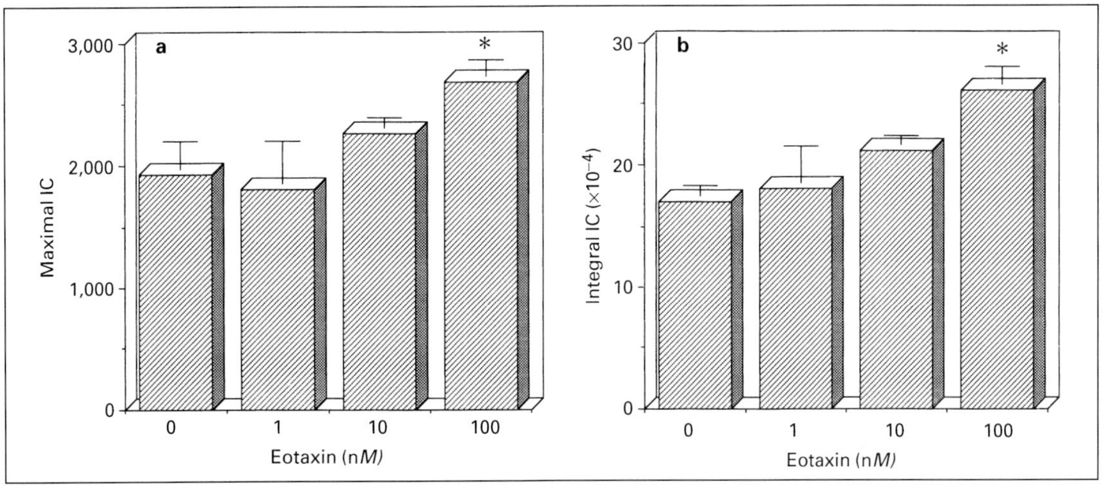

Fig. 1. A comparison of maximal IC (**a**) and integral IC (**b**) of luminol-dependent chemiluminescence to calcium ionophore A23187 in YY-1 cells treated with eotaxin (1, 10, 100 n*M*) and without eotaxin. YY-1 cells (2×10^6/ml) were precultured with or without eotaxin at 37 °C for 15 min. To the mixture of 50 µl of cells (2×10^6/ml) and 50 µl of luminol (5×10^{-4} *M*), 50 µl of calcium ionophore A23187 (final concentration 10^{-5} *M*) was added, and ROS were determined for 12 h. * $p < 0.05$ vs. values obtained from controls.

with or without an intervening amino acid between the first two cysteines [3]. In addition, recently C and CX3C chemokines families have been identified [5]. One of the CC chemokine, eotaxin was first identified as an eosinophil-specific chemoattractant in bronchoalveolar lavage fluid of an allergen-challenged model in guinea pigs [6] and has now been identified in humans [7]. Eotaxin is considered to play a key role in allergic inflammation because it is a specific chemoattractant for eosinophils. Moreover, CCR3 was identified as the specific receptor for eotaxin [8].

Chemokines induce not only chemotaxis but also activation of target cells [9]. Eotaxin is selectively chemotactic for eosinophils, but the function of eotaxin on eosinophil activation including reactive oxygen species (ROS) production has not been clarified in sufficient detail.

ROS have been considered the molecules that cause tissue injury at the inflamed site during allergic inflammation including upregulated adhesion molecule expression on inflammatory cells such as eosinophils [10]. Therefore, in this study, we examined the effect of eotaxin on ROS from YY-1 cells.

Materials and Methods

The eosinophilic subline of HL-60, YY-1, retains the physiologic properties of eosinophils, such as characteristic electron-dense granules, major basic protein, eosinophil cationic protein, and eosinophil peroxidase [11]. The production of ROS from YY-1 cells was examined with luminol-dependent chemiluminescence. YY-1 cells were preincubated at 37 °C in 5% CO_2 at 2×10^6 cells/ml in RPMI 1640 medium with serum-free condition in the presence or absence of eotaxin (1, 10, 100 n*M*; R & D Systems, USA) for 15 min, because our preliminary results revealed that the effect of eotaxin on eosinophil-oxidative metabolism was apparently observed at 15 min incubation (data not shown). To the mixture of 50 µl of eosinophils or YY-1 cells and 50 µl of luminol (5×10^{-4} *M*), 50 µl of calcium ionophore A23187 (final concentration 10^{-5} *M*) was added, and ROS in maximal intensity counts (IC) and integral IC were determined for 12 h using of ARGUS-50/2D luminometer/MP (Hamamatsu Photonics, Hamamatsu, Japan). Cell viability was maintained (95% exclusion of trypan blue dye) throughout the experiments.

Statistical Analysis

Data were expressed as mean ± SE. Differences between groups were analyzed by ANOVA; a p value ≤ 0.05 was considered significant.

Results

ROS from YY-1 cells were dose-dependently augmented by preincubation with eotaxin. While untreated eosinophils gave a maximal value of 1,928 ± 223 IC (mean ± SE, n = 4) and an integral value of 17.04 ± 1.51 IC ($\times 10^{-4}$), YY-1 cells treated with eotaxin gave a maximal value of 1,803 ± 355 IC (1 n*M*, $p > 0.05$), 2,264 ± 86 IC (10 n*M*, $p > 0.05$), 2,691 ± 124 IC (100 n*M*, $p < 0.05$) and an integral value of 18.09 ± 3.01 IC ($\times 10^{-4}$; 1 n*M*,

$p > 0.05$), 21.22 ± 0.67 IC ($\times 10^{-4}$; 10 nM, $p > 0.05$), 26.20 ± 1.41 IC ($\times 10^{-4}$; 100 nM, $p < 0.05$) (fig. 1). In other studies, eotaxin did not induce the production of ROS from YY-1 cells without calcium ionophore A23187 (data not shown).

Discussion

In this study, we investigated the possible role of eotaxin in allergic inflammation by examining eosinophil-derived ROS using the eosinophil cell line, YY-1. Eotaxin primed the production of ROS from YY-1 cells. In addition, the ROS from eosinophils showed similar results. It has been considered that ROS from eosinophils maybe one of the most important inflammatory molecules in allergic inflammation because ROS from eosinophils might injure epithelial cells at inflamed sites, resulting in airway hypersensitivity.

Eotaxin, which is a CC chemokine, was identified from bronchoalveolar lavage fluid of sensitized guinea pigs after aerosol challenge with ovalbumin, as an eosinophil chemoattractant [6]. Eotaxin showed a high and selective chemotactic activity for eosinophil. Furthermore, CCR3, a seven-transmembrane G protein-coupled receptor, was identified as a common receptor for both eotaxin and RANTES [8]. We have previously reported that RANTES not only attracts eosinophils to the inflamed site but also has activities that promote adhesion, degranulation and ROS of eosinophils, which are deeply involved in allergic inflammation [12–14]. Moreover, we demonstrated the possible elevation of RANTES in the inflamed site or plasma in the allergic diseases [15, 16].

Taking all these findings into consideration, eotaxin may play an important role in the pathogenesis of allergic inflammation through eosinophil activation by priming the eosinophil oxidative metabolism as well as being involved in selective eosinophil chemotaxis.

References

1 Bousquet J, Chanez P, Lacoste JY, Barneon G, Ghavanian N, Enander I, Venge P, Ahlstedt S, Lafontaine JS, Godard P, Michel F: Eosinophilic inflammation in asthma. N Engl J Med 1990;323:1033–1039.

2 Gleich GJ, Adolphson CR: The eosinophilic leukocyte. Adv Immunol 1986;39:177–253.

3 Marco B, Beatrice D, Bernhard M: Human chemokines: An update. Annu Rev Immunol 1997;15:675–705.

4 Murphy PM: The molecular biology of leukocyte chemoattractant receptors. Annu Rev Immunol 1994;12:593–633.

5 Bazan JF, Bacon KB, Hardiman G, Wang W, Soo K, Rossi D, Greaves DR, Zlotnik A, Schall TJ: A new class of membrane-bound chemokine with a CX3C motif. Nature 1997;385: 640–644.

6 Jose PJ, Johnson DA, Collins PD, Walsh DT, Moqbel R, Totty NF, Truong O, Hsuan JJ, Williams TJ: Eotaxin: A potent eosinophil chemoattractant cytokine detected in a guinea pig model of allergic airways inflammation. J Exp Med 1994;179:881–887.

7 Ponath PD, Qin S, Ringler DJ, Lewise IC, Wang J, Kassam N, Smith H, Shi X, Gonzalo JA, Newman W, Ramos J, Mackay CR: Cloning of the human eosinophil chemoattractant, eotaxin. J Clin Invest 1996;97:604–612.

8 Kitaura M, Nakajima T, Imai T, Harada S, Combadiere C, Tiffany HL, Murphy PM, Yoshie O: Molecular cloning of human eotaxin, an eosinophil-selective CC chemokine, and identification of a specific eosinophil eotaxin receptor, CC chemokine receptor 3. J Biol Chem 1996;271:7725–7730.

9 Alam R, Stafford S, Forsythe P, Harrison R, Faubion D, Lett-Brown MA, Grant JA: RANTES is a chemotactic and activating factor for human eosinophils. J Immunol 1993; 150:3442–3447.

10 Chihara J, Kakazu T, Higasimoto I, Yamamoto T, Kurachi D, Nakajima S: Increased eosinophil oxidative metabolism by treatment with soluble intercellular adhesion molecule-1. Int Arch Allergy Immunol 1995;108(suppl 1):45–47.

11 Hori K, Hirashima M, Ueno M, Matsuda M, Waga S, Tsurufuji S, Yodoi J: Regulation of eosinophil migration by adult T cell leukemia-derived factor. J Immunol 1993;151:5624–5630.

12 Chihara J, Yamada H, Yamamoto T, Kurachi D, Hayashi N, Kayaba H, Urayama O: Priming effect of RANTES on eosinophil oxidative metabolism. Allergy 1998;53:1178–1182.

13 Kakazu T, Chihara J, Saito A, Higashimoto I, Yamamoto T, Kurachi D, Nakajima S: Effect of RANTES on intracellular expression of EG2 antigen in eosinophil. Int Arch Allergy Immunol 1995;108(suppl 1):43–44.

14 Kakazu T, Chihara J, Saito A, Nakajima S: Effect of RANTES on eosinophil adhesion to plates coated with recombinant soluble intercellular adhesion molecule-1 and expression of β2-integrin adhesion molecules on eosinophils. Int Arch Allergy Immunol 1995;108(suppl 1): 9–11.

15 Chihara J, Yamada H, Takamura E, Yoshino K, Nakajima S: Possible presence of RANTES in tears of patients with allergic conjunctivitis. Int Arch Allergy Immunol 1995;106:428.

16 Chihara J, Yasuba H, Tsuda A, Urayama O, Saito N, Honda K, Kayaba H, Yamasita T, Kurimoto F, Yamada H: Elevation of the plasma level of RANTES during asthma attacks. J Allergy Clin Immunol 1997;100:S52–55.

International Archives of Allergy and Immunology

Int Arch Allergy Immunol 1999;120(suppl 1):51–53

Intracellular Signaling Pathways in Human Eosinophil Activation: Role of a β_2 Integrin, $\alpha_M\beta_2$

Masahiko Kato[a] Hirokazu Kimura[b] Atsushi Tachibana[a] Youichi Motegi[a] Kenichi Tokuyama[a] Hirohito Kita[c] Akihiro Morikawa[a]

[a]Department of Pediatrics, Gunma University School of Medicine, [b]Gunma Prefectural Institute of Public Health and Environmental Sciences, Maebashi, Gunma, Japan; [c]Department of Immunology and Internal Medicine, Mayo Clinic and Foundation, Rochester, Minn., USA

Key Words
Eosinophil · Integrin · Adhesion · Signal transduction · Superoxide

Abstract
Cellular adhesion is crucial roles for eosinophil effector functions such as degranulation. Here, we focused on the role of a β_2 integrin, $\alpha_M\beta_2$, in intracellular signaling pathways of human eosinophil activation. We found that the ligation of $\alpha_M\beta_2$ triggers the activation of an intracellular signaling cascade, including protein tyrosine phosphorylation and phosphoinositide turnover, and subsequent cellular degranulation in human eosinophils. These signaling events may play important roles in adhesion-dependent cellular functions of eosinophils.

Eosinophils are recognized as a proinflammatory granulocyte implicated in host immunity to parasite infections and allergic diseases such as bronchial asthma, allergic rhinitis, and atopic dermatitis [1]. Appropriate stimuli such as immunoglobulins induce degranulation of toxic eosinophil granule proteins, including eosinophil-derived neurotoxin, major basic protein, eosinophil cationic protein, and eosinophil peroxidase [2]. Subsequently, the tissue damages induced by these eosinophilic granule proteins and oxygen radicals contribute to airway inflammation associated with such diseases [1]. However, at present, the details and underlying signal transduction mechanisms for effector functions of eosinophils remain to be elucidated.

Cell adhesion is a crucial step for activation of inflammatory cells [3]. Evidence suggests that adhesion molecules, such as $\alpha_4\beta_1$ (VLA-4, CD49d/CD29) and $\alpha_M\beta_2$ (Mac-1, CD11b/CD18), play an important role in eosinophil recruitment into the sites of inflammation in allergic disease. These integrins, particularly β_2 integrin, modulate eosinophil activation, such as degranulation and superoxide anion generation, with various physiologic stimuli [4]. Previously, we and others showed that eosinophil adhesion through β_2 integrin is a crucial step for degranulation of eosinophils [5–8]. For example, eosinophil degranulation induced by IgG immobilized onto tissue culture plates or Sepharose beads was inhibited by anti-CD18 (β_2 integrin) monoclonal antibody (mAb) [5]. Further, cell adhesion mediated by $\alpha_M\beta_2$ strikingly influenced the degranulation response of the eosinophils triggered by a lipid mediator, platelet-activating factor (PAF), and by a cytokine, granulocyte macrophage colony-stimulating factor [6], or interleukin (IL)-5 [8]. The ability of these secre-

KARGER
Fax + 41 61 306 12 34
E-Mail karger@karger.ch
www.karger.com

1018–2438/99/1205–0051$17.50/0

Accessible online at:
http://BioMedNet.com/karger

Dr. Masahiko Kato
Department of Pediatrics, Gunma University School of Medicine
3-39-22 Showa-machi
Maebashi, Gunma 371-8511 (Japan)

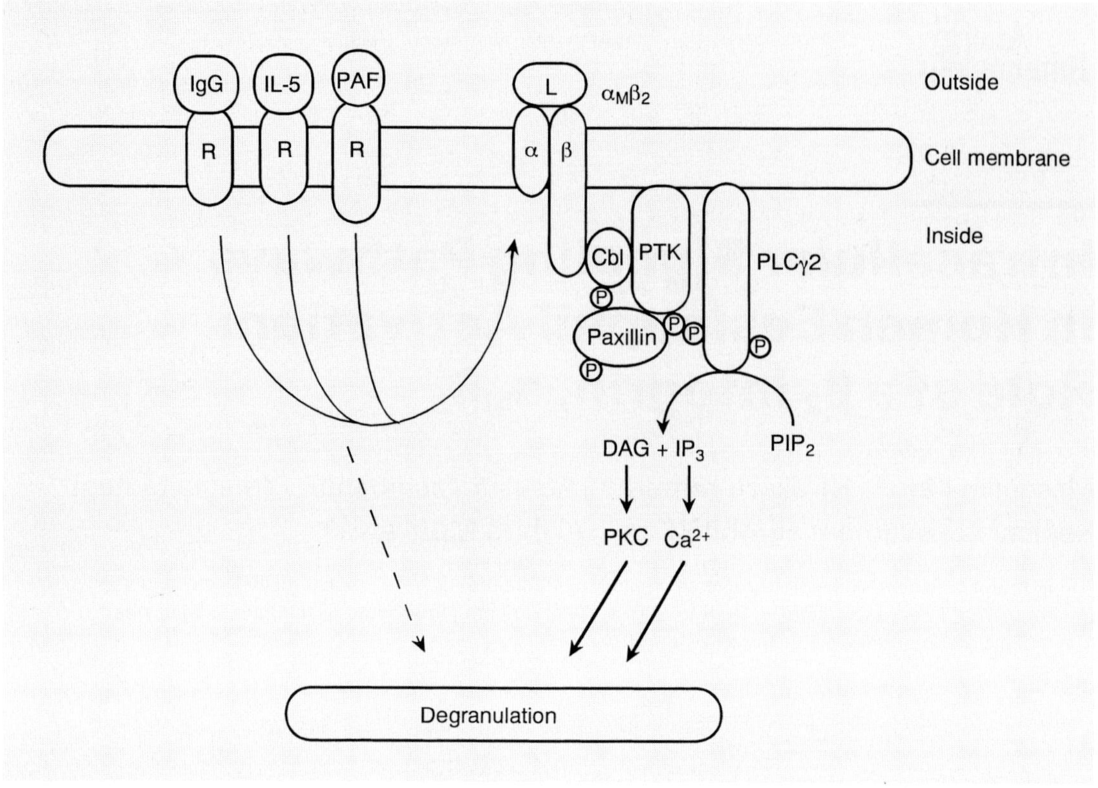

Fig. 1. Signal transduction in human eosinophil activation through $a_M\beta_2$. L = Ligand; R = receptor; P = tyrosine phosphorylation; Ig = immunoglobulins; Cbl = the product of c-*cbl* protooncogene; PLC = phospholipase C; PTK = protein tyrosine kinase; PIP_2 = phosphatidylinositol-4,5-bisphosphate; IP_3 = inositol-1,4,5-triphosphate; DAG = diacylglycerol; PKC = protein kinase C.

tagogues to induce eosinophil degranulation was minimal when cells were kept in suspension. Interestingly, extracellular matrix proteins, such as laminin and fibronectin, which bind to eosinophils in a β_1 integrin-dependent manner, interfered with β_2 integrin-mediated adhesion and concomitantly inhibited eosinophil degranulation induced by PAF, the complement fragment C5a, or IL-5 [9].

Recently, we studied the role of $\alpha_M\beta_2$ on superoxide anion (O_2^-) generation stimulated by PAF. The O_2^- generation was assayed by a highly sensitive and specific chemiluminescence method using a *Cypridina* luciferin analog as the amplifier [10]. We found that PAF induced 5 times the amount of O_2^- generation in human eosinophils compared with that in human neutrophils when cells adhered to albumin-coated tubes. This increased O_2^- generation in eosinophils was completely inhibited when cells were kept in suspension and almost completely blocked by the pretreatment of anti-CD18 mAb. Although phorbol myristate acetate, a direct protein kinase C activator, induced larger amounts of O_2^- generation from eosinophils compared with PAF, this increased O_2^- generation was not affected by the treatment of stirring the cell suspension and of anti-CD18 mAb. These results confirm the important role of $\alpha_M\beta_2$ in effector functions of eosinophils induced by a membrane receptor stimulator such as PAF.

Based on these observations and our results, as shown in figure 1, we propose a signaling model of membrane-receptor-induced eosinophil activation such as degranulation and O_2^- generation. The PAF receptor has a seven transmembrane domain and is thought to be coupled to the pertussis toxin-sensitive GTP-binding protein (Gi protein) [11]. On the other hand, the IL-5 receptor consists of a heterodimeric α and β common chain, and the IgG receptor is identified as FcγRII in human eosinophils. Although the construction of these receptors and their accessory signaling molecules were different from those of PAF, both of receptor-mediated stimulations induce the CD11b expression on eosinophil surface and the conformational change of integrin molecules. This process is the so-called 'inside-out' signaling similarly seen in lymphocytes [12]. Once the clustering or multimerization of $\alpha_M\beta_2$ at the sites of focal adhesion occurs, the 'outside-in' signal is triggered into the cells [12]. Recently, we have shown that the engagement of $\alpha_M\beta_2$ induced tyrosine phosphorylation of several proteins including an unidentified 115-kD protein, the product of c-*cbl* protooncogene, Cbl, and paxillin, a cytoskeletal protein. Furthermore, this stimulation of $\alpha_M\beta_2$ increased the production of inositol phosphates, and subsequently triggered the degranulation of eosinophils [8]. These findings collectively indicate that $\alpha_M\beta_2$ plays a crucial role not only in cell adhesion but also in effector functions of eosinophils. This $\alpha_M\beta_2$-mediated activation of eosinophils may be particularly important in the pathophysiology of eosinophilic diseases and allergic inflammation, in which various types of cells show an increased expression of ligands for $\alpha_M\beta_2$, as typified by ICAM-1 expression by bronchial epithelial cells in bronchial asthma [13].

Indeed, $\alpha_M\beta_2$ is implicated in the degranulation of eosinophils and the development of bronchial hyperresponsiveness in cynomolgus monkeys challenged with allergen as a model of human bronchial asthma [14]. Therefore, although analyses of the detailed molecular mechanisms leading to the activation of eosinophils following the engagement of $\alpha_M\beta_2$ are still under way, the identification of several key molecules in the signaling pathway would provide an insight into integrin-mediated transmembrane signaling and possibly open new avenues for the treatment of patients with eosinophilia and allergic diseases such as bronchial asthma.

References

1 Butterfield JH, Leiferman KM, Gleich GJ: Eosinophil-associated diseases; in Frank MM, Austen KF, Claman HN, Unanue ER (eds): Samuter's Immunologic Diseases. Boston, Little, Brownand, 1995, pp 501–527.

2 Butterworth AE, Remold HG, Houba V, David JR, Franks D, David PH, Sturrock RF: Antibody-dependent eosinophil-mediated damage to ^{51}Cr-labeled schistosomula of *Schistosoma mansoni:* Mediation by IgG, and inhibition by antigen-antibody complexes. J Immunol 1977; 118:2230–2236.

3 Springer TA: Adhesion receptors of the immune system. Nature 1990;346:425–434.

4 Hartnell A, Moqbel R, Walsh GM, Bradley B, Kay AB: Fcγ and CD11/CD18 receptor expression on normal density and low density human eosinophils. Immunology 1990;69:264–270.

5 Kaneko M, Horie S, Kato M, Gleich GJ, Kita H: A crucial role for β_2 integrin in the activation of eosinophils stimulated by IgG. J Immunol 1995;155:2631–2641.

6 Horie S, Kita H: CD11b/CD18 (Mac-1) is required for degranulation of human eosinophils induced by human recombinant granulocyte-macrophage colony-stimulating factor and platelet-activating factor. J Immunol 1994;152: 5427–5467.

7 Laudanna C, Melotti P, Bonizzato C, Piacentini G, Boner A, Serra MC, Berton G: Ligation of members of the β_1 or the β_2 subfamilies of integrins by antibodies triggers eosinophil respiratory burst and spreading. Immunology 1993;80:273–280.

8 Kato M, Abraham RT, Okada S, Kita H: Ligation of the β_2 integrin triggers activation and degranulation of human eosinophils. Am J Respir Cell Mol Biol 1998;18:675–686.

9 Kita H, Horie S, Gleich GJ: Extracellular matrix proteins attenuate activation and degranulation of stimulated eosinophils. J Immunol 1996;156:1174–1181.

10 Kato M, Tokuyama K, Morikawa A, Kuroume T, Barnes PJ: Platelet-activating factor-induced enhancement of superoxide anion generation in guinea pigs. Eur J Pharmacol 1993; 232:7–12.

11 Nakamura M, Honda Z, Izumi T, Sakanaka C, Mutoh H, Minami M, Bito H, Sayama Y, Matsumoto T, Noma M, Simizu T: Molecular cloning and expression of platelet-activating factor receptor from human leukocytes. J Biol Chem 1991;266:20400–20405.

12 Lub M, van Kooyk Y, Fridor CG: Ins and outs of LFA-1. Immunol Today 1995;16:479–483.

13 Canonica GW, Ciprandi G, Pesce GP, Buscaglia S, Paolieri F, Bagnasco M: ICAM-1 on epithelial cells in allergic subjects: A hallmark of allergic inflammation. Int Arch Allergy Immunol 1995;107:99–102.

14 Wegner CD, Gundel R, Churchill L, Letts LG: Adhesion glycoproteins as regulators of airway inflammation: Emphasis on the role of ICAM-1; in Holgate ST, Austen KF, Lichtenstein LM, Kay AB (eds): Asthma: Physiology, Immunopharmacology, and Treatment. London, Academic Press, 1993, pp 227–241.

International Archives of
Allergy and
Immunology

Int Arch Allergy Immunol 1999;120(suppl 1):54–59

Tumor Necrosis Factor-α Mediates Antiapoptotic Signals Partially via p38 MAP Kinase Activation in Human Eosinophils

Kayo Tsukahara Atsuhito Nakao Masaki Hiraguri Satoshi Miike
Mizuko Mamura Yasushi Saito Itsuo Iwamoto

Department of Internal Medicine II, Chiba University School of Medicine, Chiba, Japan

Key Words
Eosinophil apoptosis · Tumor necrosis factor-α · p38 MAP kinase

Abstract
Tumor necrosis factor-α (TNF-α) is a proinflammatory cytokine with many biological effects on a variety of cells. In particular, TNF-α has been shown to act as a death or survival factor which mediates apoptosis or antiapoptotic signals in various types of cells. In eosinophils, TNF-α has been reported to activate eosinophil functions. However, it is not clearly defined whether TNF-α delivers antiapoptotic signals in eosinophils. In order to determine whether TNF-α prevents eosinophil apoptosis, we examined the effect of TNF-α on eosinophil apoptosis by the survival assay and cell cycle analysis. We also determined whether intracellular MAP kinases (ERKs, Jun kinase/JNK, and p38 MAP kinase) are involved in the TNF-α-induced signaling for the prevention of eosinophil apoptosis. We showed that TNF-α mediated antiapoptotic signals in human eosinophils in part via activation of p38 MAP kinase, but not via activation of ERKs and JNK. Our data suggest that TNF-α/p38 MAP kinase pathways are involved in the regulation of eosinophil survival and, thus, would be important for the development of allergic eosinophil-rich inflammation.

Introduction

Tumor necrosis factor-α (TNF-α) is a proinflammatory cytokine with many biological effects on a variety of cells [1]. In eosinophils, TNF-α enhances eosinophil cytotoxic activity against parasites [2], directly induces the release of chemical mediators [3], and mediates recruitment of eosinophils into the airways [4]. These findings suggest that TNF-α regulates activation of eosinophil functions. Since eosinophils are major effector cells for allergic inflammation [5], these data suggest that TNF-α plays a certain role in allergic inflammation. In agreement with the findings, TNF-α production was reported to be increased in the airways of asthmatics [6].

Cytokines such as GM-CSF transmit antiapoptotic signals in eosinophils and are involved in blood and tissue eosinophilia, which is important for the development of allergic inflammation [7]. However, although TNF-α is well known to act as a cytokine which regulates cell death [8], it is not clearly defined whether TNF-α delivers antiapoptotic signals in eosinophils. To clarify the issue, we decided to determine whether TNF-α prevents eosinophil apoptosis and, if so, how TNF-α delivers antiapoptotic signals in eosinophils. For this purpose, we examined the effect of TNF-α on eosinophil apoptosis and the activation of intracellular MAP kinases (ERKs, Jun kinase/JNK, and p38 MAP kinase) of eosinophils. We also stud-

KARGER
Fax + 41 61 306 12 34
E-Mail karger@karger.ch
www.karger.com

1018–2438/99/1205–0054$17.50/0

Accessible online at:
http://BioMedNet.com/karger

Itsuo Iwamoto, MD
Department of Internal Medicine II, Chiba University School of Medicine
1-8-1 Inohana, Chiba City, Chiba 260-8670 (Japan)
Tel. +81 43 226 2090, Fax +81 43 226 2095
E-Mail iwamoto@intmed02.m.chiba-u.ac.jp

ied the effect of a specific inhibitor of p38 MAP kinase SB203580 on the TNF-α-induced signaling for the prevention of eosinophil apoptosis.

We showed here that TNF-α mediated antiapoptotic signals in human eosinophils in part via activation of p38 MAP kinase, but not via activation of ERKs and JNK. Our data suggest that TNF-α/p38 MAP kinase pathways are involved in the regulation of eosinophil survival and, thus, would be important for the development of allergic inflammation. Therefore, manipulation of TNF-α/p38 MAP kinase pathways might be useful for treatment of allergic inflammation.

Materials and Methods

Culture and Survival Assay of Eosinophils

Human eosinophils were purified from heparinized venous blood of healthy individuals by Percoll density gradient centrifugation and a magnetic cell sorting using MACS anti-CD16 microbeads as described by Hansel et al. [9]. Pure eosinophils (purity >98%) were obtained by CD16-negative selection and suspended in Hanks' balanced salt solution.

Eosinophils (purity 98–100%, viability >99%) were cultured in triplicate with or without recombinant human TNF-α (5×10^4 IU/ml; Pepro Tech, London, UK) or recombinant human GM-CSF (10^{-12} *M*; Kirin, Tokyo, Japan) in RPMI 1640 medium containing 10% fetal calf serum (FCS) in 24-well plates (1×10^5 cells/well) for 1–4 days at 37°C in a humidified atmosphere of 5% CO_2 in air. These cultures were also performed in the presence or absence of anti-GM-CSF antibody (10 µg/ml; R & D Systems, Minneapolis, Minn., USA). In some experiments, cells were incubated with TNF-α (5×10^4 IU/ml) in the presence or absence of 5 µ*M* SB203580 (SmithKline Beecham), a specific inhibitor of p38 MAP kinase [10].

After the culture, cells were suspended in phosphate-buffered saline containing 1% FCS, stained with trypan blue solution, and counted with hemocytometer. Stained cells were counted as dead cells.

Determination of Eosinophil Apoptosis

Apoptosis of eosinophils was assessed by the cell cycle analysis assay [11]. After 4 days of culture, eosinophils were fixed with cold 80% ethanol, washed and resuspended in a permeability buffer (0.1 m*M* EDTA and 0.1% Triton X-100 in PBS) containing RNAase (25 µg/ml). Then, cells were stained with 50 µg/ml propidium iodide at 4°C in the dark overnight, and the propidium iodide fluorescence of individual nuclei was analyzed by FACScan (Becton Dickinson, Mountain View, Calif., USA). Cells with hypodiploid DNA were counted as apoptotic cells.

Immunoblotting

Phosphorylation of ERKs (ERK1 and ERK2) was determined by SDS-PAGE and Western blotting using anti-MAP kinase antibody (erk1-CT; Upstate Biotechnology, Lake Placid, N.Y., USA) as previously reported [12]. Phosphorylation (or activation) of p38 MAP kinase and JNK/SAPK was measured by using a p38 MAPK assay kit and a JNK/SAPK assay kit (New England Biolabs, Beverly, Mass., USA) according to the manufacturer's instruction.

Data Analysis

Data are summarized as mean ± SD. The statistical analysis of the results was performed by the paired t test. p values <0.05 were considered significant.

Results

TNF-α Mediates Antiapoptotic Signals in Human Eosinophils

To determine whether TNF-α affects eosinophil apoptosis, we examined the effect of TNF-α on the viability of eosinophils collected from peripheral blood of healthy donors. It has been shown that mature eosinophils die of apoptosis in a couple of days in the absence of survival factors such as GM-CSF [13], and we confirmed the findings (survival rate at 96 h; medium alone 11.7 ± 2.9% vs. 10^{-12} *M* GM-CSF 72.9 ± 8.0%, mean ± SD, n = 4 experiments, $p < 0.001$; fig. 1a).

TNF-α (5.0×10^4 IU/ml) significantly increased the viability of eosinophils compared with the control (survival rate at 96 h; 49.8 ± 7.3%, n = 4, $p < 0.02$) (fig. 1a). In addition, we found the dose-dependent increase of eosinophil viability by TNF-α at the concentration of 0.5×10^4, 1.0×10^4 and 5.0×10^4 IU/ml (data not shown). Furthermore, we found that incubation of eosinophils with TNF-α (5.0×10^4 IU/ml) led to a reduction of the hypodiploid peak in human eosinophils (fig. 1b). These data indicated that TNF-α prevented eosinophil apoptosis, suggesting that TNF-α mediated antiapoptotic signals in human eosinophils.

GM-CSF Is Not Involved in Antiapoptotic Signals of TNF-α in Eosinophils

Since we found that TNF-α prevented eosinophil apoptosis and TNF-α-induced GM-CSF production in eosinophils was implicated [14], we sought to determine whether the effect of TNF-α on eosinophil survival was a secondary effect via TNF-α-induced production of GM-CSF. For this purpose, we examined the effect of anti-GM-CSF antibody on TNF-α-mediated eosinophil survival. As shown in figure 2, the antibody against GM-CSF (10 µg/ml) did not affect TNF-α-induced inhibition of eosinophil apoptosis (survival rate at 96 h; TNF-α 52.2 ± 7.7% vs. TNF-α + anti-GM-CSF antibody 54.4 ± 5.8%, n = 3), whereas the antibody completely blocked GM-CSF-induced inhibition of eosinophil apoptosis (survival rate at 96 h; GM-CSF 80.5 ± 6.2% vs. GM-CSF + anti-GM-CSF antibody 32.0 ± 6.8%, n = 3, $p < 0.05$). The anti-GM-CSF antibody alone did not affect the viability of eosinophils (survival rate at 96 h; medium alone 17.1

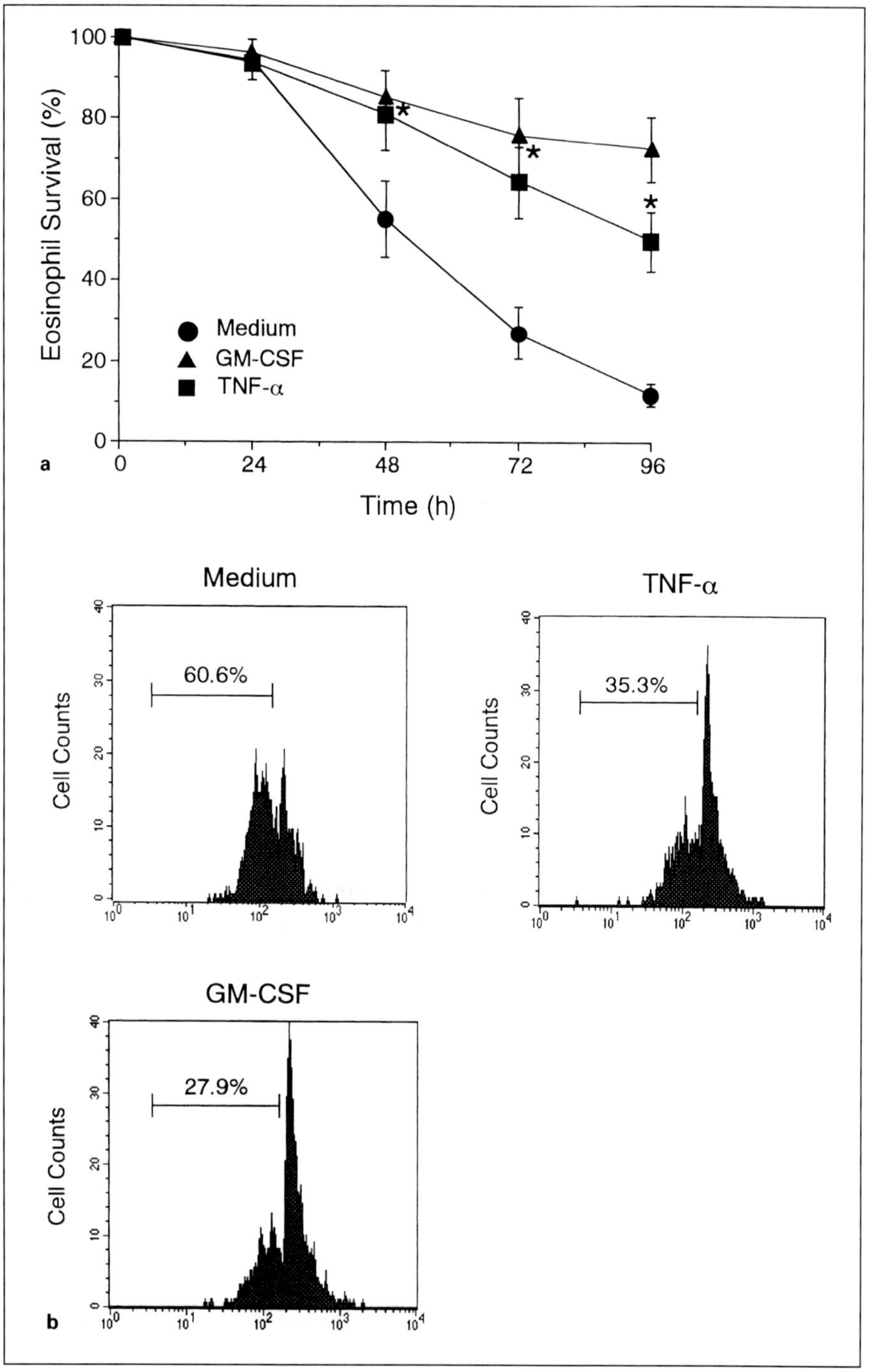

Fig. 1. Effect of TNF-α on apoptosis in human eosinophils. Human eosinophils were cultured with or without TNF-α (5.0×10^4 IU/ml) or GM-CSF (10^{-12} *M*) in 24-well plates (1×10^5 cells/well) at 37 °C for 1–4 days. After the culture, the cell viability was assessed every 24 h by counting cells with trypan blue solution (**a**). Data are means ± SD for four experiments at each time point. *$p < 0.02$ vs. mean value of the corresponding control response (medium alone). The data of eosinophil apoptosis detected by the cell cycle analysis (**b**) are representative of three experiments.

± 4.3% vs. medium + anti-GM-CSF antibody 26.1 ± 5.8%, n = 3) (fig. 2). These findings indicated that the effect of TNF-α on eosinophils was not secondary by GM-CSF production, suggesting that TNF-α mediated anti-apoptotic signals in human eosinophils as a primary biological effect.

TNF-α Mediates Antiapoptotic Signals in Part via p38 MAP Kinase Activation in Eosinophils

Intracellular pathways of TNF receptors are either linked with apoptosis, NF-κB translocation, and activation of MAP kinases (ERKs, JNK and p38 MAP kinase) [15–19]. However, the role of these pathways in TNF-α-

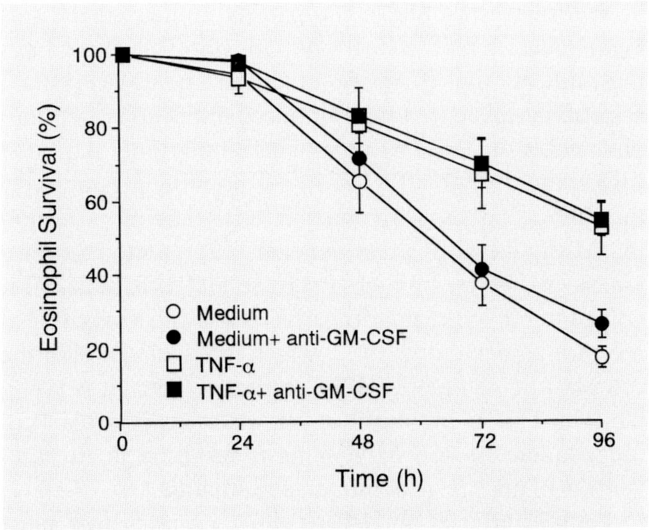

Fig. 2. Effect of anti-GM-CSF antibody on TNF-α-induced inhibition of apoptosis in human eosinophils. Eosinophils were cultured with TNF-α (5.0 × 10^4 IU/ml) for 1–4 days in the presence or absence of anti-GM-CSF antibody (10 μg/ml), and the cell viability was assessed every 24 h counting cells with trypan blue solution. Data are means ± SD for three experiments at each time point.

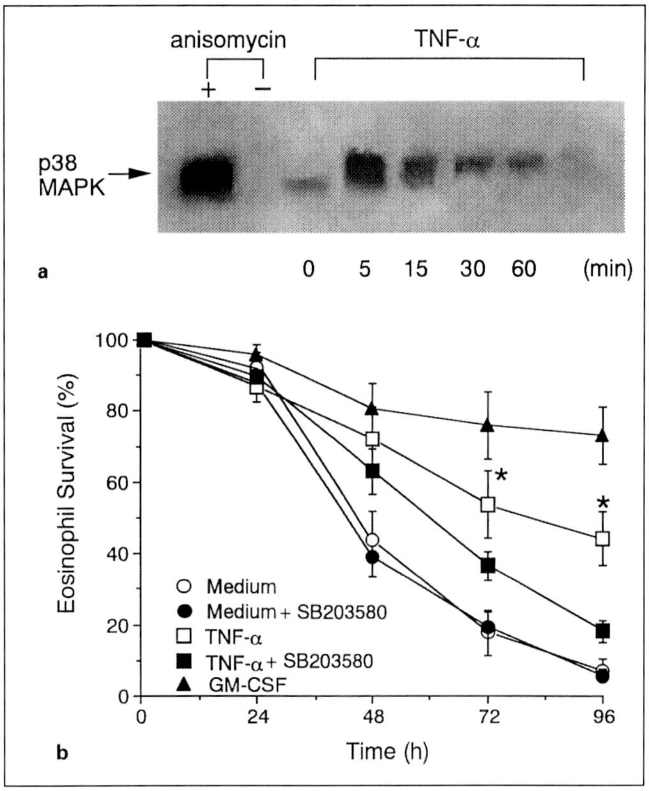

Fig. 3. Effect of TNF-α on p38 MAP kinase phosphorylation (**a**) and effect of SB203580 on TNF-α-induced inhibition of apoptosis (**b**) in human eosinophils. **a** Eosinophils (5 × 10^5/ml) were stimulated with TNF-α (5.0 × 10^4 IU/ml) at 37°C for 5–60 min. Cell lysates were then subjected to Western blotting as described in Methods. The position of phosphorylated p38 MAP kinase at approximately 38 kD is shown by the arrow. Controls were C6 cell extracts with or without treatment of anisomycin (1 μ*M* for 10 min). The data are representative of three experiments. **b** Eosinophils were cultured with TNF-α (5.0 × 10^4 IU/ml) for 1–4 days in the presence or absence of SB203580 (5 μ*M*), and the cell viability was assessed every 24 h by counting cells with trypan blue solution. Data are means ± SD of three experiments at each time point. * $p < 0.05$ vs. mean value of the corresponding response (TNF-α alone).

induced inhibition of eosinophil apoptosis has not been defined. Thus, we decided to determine whether these pathways are involved in TNF-α-induced inhibition of eosinophil apoptosis. In particular, we focused on the role of MAP kinase in the TNF-α-mediated signaling since MAP kinases are essential for diverse signal transduction pathways [20].

We first determined whether TNF-α activated MAP kinases (ERKs, JNK and p38 MAP kinase) in human eosinophils. Western blotting analysis showed that TNF-α phosphorylated p38 MAP kinase in eosinophils (fig. 3a). However, we did not find any phosphorylation of ERKs (ERK1 and ERK2) and JNK in eosinophils after stimulation of TNF-α (data not shown). The p38 MAP kinase phosphorylation in eosinophils reached a peak at 5 min, with a gradual decline until 60 min after stimulation of TNF-α (fig. 3a). These findings indicated that p38 MAP kinase was activated by TNF-α in eosinophils. Therefore, to further determine whether the activation of p38 MAP kinase by TNF-α is involved in TNF-α-induced inhibition of eosinophil apoptosis, we examined the effect of SB203580, a selective inhibitor of p38 MAP kinase [10], on TNF-α-induced inhibition of eosinophil apoptosis. As shown in figure 3b, SB203580 (5 μ*M*) inhibited the survival effect of TNF-α in eosinophils by 59% (survival rate at 96 h; TNF-α 44.0 ± 7.3% vs. TNF-α + SB203580 18.2 ± 3.0%, n = 3, $p < 0.05$). SB203580 itself was not cytotoxic to eosinophils (fig. 3b) and the effect of SB203580 was dose-dependent (data not shown). These findings indicated that activation of p38 MAP kinase was partially involved in TNF-α-induced inhibition of eosinophil apoptosis.

Discussion

Prevention of eosinophil apoptosis by cytokines such as GM-CSF has been well characterized and is involved in tissue and blood eosinophilia, which is important for allergic inflammation [13]. Although TNF-α has also been suggested to play a certain role in allergic inflammation and TNF-α is well known to act as a regulator of cell survival [8], it has not been clearly defined whether TNF-α is involved in the prevention of eosinophil apoptosis. Our findings (fig. 1, 2) clearly indicate that TNF-α prevents eosinophil apoptosis as a primary effect. Thus, we conclude that TNF-α is one of the cytokines which act to prevent eosinophil apoptosis. TNF-α may cooperate with other cytokines in the development of allergic eosinophil-rich inflammation.

TNF-α binds to two ubiquitously expressed receptors, TNF receptor I (TNFRI/p55) and TNF receptor II (TNFRII/p75), which do not share any homology within their cytoplasmic domains [15]. Intracellular pathways originating at the TNF receptors are either linked with apoptosis, NF-κB translocation, or activation of MAP kinases (ERKs, JNK and p38 MAP kinase) [15–19]. Previous studies have shown that intracellular pathways delivering TNF-α-induced inhibition of apoptosis depend on cell types and cellular context [15]. Our data indicated that TNF-α-induced inhibition of eosinophil apoptosis involved in p38 MAP kinase pathways, which is in agreement with the recent findings in a murine fibroblast cell line by Roulston et al. [21]. In addition, Beyaert et al. [22] reported that p38 MAP kinase was a crucial mediator in TNF-induced activation of NF-κB-dependent gene expression. Recent studies have suggested that NF-κB plays a key role for prevention of apoptosis [23–25]. In eosinophils, involvement of Raf-1 kinase, which may lie upstream of NF-κB, in IL-5-induced antiapoptotic signals was recently suggested by Pazdrak et al. [26]. Thus, it is possible that p38 MAP kinase might act upstream of NF-κB and prevents apoptosis by inducing NF-κB activation in human eosinophils. We are investigating the role of NF-κB in the prevention of eosinophil apoptosis by TNF-α.

We found that SB203580 partially inhibited the survival effect of TNF-α in eosinophils (fig. 3b). These findings indicate that pathways other than p38 MAP kinase are also involved in TNF-α-induced inhibition of eosinophil apoptosis. Since we did not detect phosphorylation of ERKs and JNK by TNF-α in eosinophils, it is unlikely that ERKs or JNK is involved in the antiapoptotic signaling. Most recently, Carpentier et al. [19] reported that two kinase pathways, p38 MAP kinase and IκB kinase, involved in NF-κB regulation, diverged at the level of TNF receptor-associated factor 2, which is associated with the cytoplasmic segment of TNF receptors. Thus, it is possible that TNF-α may induce NF-κB activation via IκB, independent of p38 MAP kinase, resulting in the prevention of apoptosis in human eosinophils.

Levi-Schaffer et al. [14] recently suggested that mast cell-derived TNF-α enhanced eosinophil survival by inducing GM-CSF production from eosinophils, which may be inconsistent with our findings that TNF-α directly affects eosinophil survival (fig. 2). However, they used mast cell/eosinophil coculture or mast cell sonicates to stimulate eosinophils. In the system they used, one cannot exclude the influence of factors (other than TNF-α) to induce GM-CSF production from eosinophils, which may explain the discrepancy.

In summary, we have shown that TNF-α mediates antiapoptotic signals in human eosinophils possibly in part via activation of p38 MAP kinase. Our data suggest that manipulation of TNF-α/p38 MAP kinase pathways might be useful for the treatment of allergic eosinophil-rich inflammation.

Acknowledgments

This work was supported in part by grants from the Ministry of Education, Science and Culture, Japan.

References

1 Tracey K, Cerami A: Tumor necrosis factor, other cytokines and disease. Annu Rev Cell Biol 1993;9:317–343.
2 Silberstein DS, David JR: Tumor necrosis factor enhances eosinophil toxicity to *Schistosoma mansoni* larvae. Proc Natl Acad Sci USA 1986; 83:1055–1059.
3 Horie S, Gleich GJ, Kita H: Cytokines directly induce degranulation and superoxide production from human eosinophils. J Allergy Clin Immunol 1996;98:371–381.
4 Lukacs NW, Strieter RM, Chenusue SW, Widmer M, Kunkel SL: TNF-α mediates recruitment of neutrophils and eosinophils during airway inflammation. J Immunol 1995; 154:5411–5417.
5 Gleich GJ: The eosinophil and bronchial asthma: Current understanding. J Allergy Clin Immunol 1990;85:422–436.
6 Cembryznska-Nowak M, Szklarz E, Inglot AD, Teodoczyk-Injeyan JA: Elevated release of tumor necrosis factor-α and interferon-γ by bronchoalveolar leukocytes from patients with bronchial asthma. Am Rev Respir Dis 1993; 147:291–296.
7 Simon H-U, Yousefi S, Schranz C, Schapowal A, Bachert C, Blase K: Direct demonstration of delayed eosinophil apoptosis as a mechanism causing tissue eosinophilia. J Immunol 1997; 158:3902–3908.

8 Van Antwerp DJ, Martin SJ, Verma IM, Green DR: Inhibition of TNF-induced apoptosis by NF-κB. Trends Cell Biol 1998;8:107–111.
9 Hansel TT, De Vries IJM, Iff T, Rihs S, Wandzilak M, Betz S, Blaser K, Walker C: An improved immunomagnetic procedure for the isolation of highly purified human blood eosinophils. J Immunol Methods 1991;145:105–110.
10 Cuend A, Rouse J, Doza YN, Neier R, Cohen P, Gallagher TF, Young RR, Lee JC: SB203580 is a specific inhibitor of a MAP kinase homologue which is stimulated by cellular stresses and interleukin-1. FEBS Lett 1995;364:229–233.
11 Nicoletti I, Migliorati G, Pagliacci MC, Grignani F, Riccardi C: A rapid and simple method for measuring thymocyte apoptosis by propidium iodide staining and flow cytometry. J Immunol Methods 1991;139:271–279.
12 Hiraguri M, Miike S, Sano H, Kurasawa K, Saito Y, Iwamoto I: Granulocyte-macrophage colony-stimulating factor and interleukin-5 activate mitogen-activated protein kinase through Jak2 kinase and phosphatidylinositol 3-kinase in human eosinophils. J Allergy Clin Immunol 1997;100:S45–51.
13 Simon HU, Yousefi S, Fibbert B, Levi-Schaffer F, Blaser K: Anti-apoptotic signals of granulocyte-macrophage colony-stimulating factor are transduced via Jak2 tyrosine kinase in eosinophils. Eur J Immunol 1997;27:3536–3539.
14 Levi-Schaffer F, Temkin V, Malamud V, Feld S, Zilberman Y: Mast cells enhance eosinophil survival in vitro: Role of TNF-α and granulocyte-macrophage colony stimulating factor. J Immunol 1998;160:5554–5562.
15 Tewari M, Dixit VM: Signaling through members of the tumor necrosis factor receptor family; in Heldin C-H, Purton M (eds): Signal Transduction. London, Chapman & Hall, 1996, pp 79–92.
16 Liu Z-G, Hsu H, Goeddel DV, Karin M: Dissection of TNF receptor I effector functions: JNK activation it not linked to apoptosis while NF-κB activation prevents cell death. Cell 1996;87:565–576.
17 Natoli G, Costanzo A, Ianni A, Templeton DJ, Woodgett JR, Balsano C, Levrero M: Activation of SAPK/JNK by TNF receptor I through a noncytotoxic TRAF2-dependent pathway. Science 1997;275:200–203.
18 Cesaris PD, Starace D, Riccioli A, Padula F, Filippini A, Ziparo E: Tumor necrosis factor-α induces interleukin-6 production and integrin ligand expression by distinct transduction pathways. J Biol Chem 1998;27:7566–7571.
19 Carpentier I, Declercq W, Malinin NL, Wallach D, Fiers W, Beyaert R: TRAF2 plays a dual role in NF-κB-dependent gene activation by mediating the TNF-induced activation of p38 MAPK and IkB kinase pathways. FEBS Lett 1998;425:195–198.
20 Nishida E, Gotoh Y: The MAP kinase cascade is essential for diverse signal transduction pathways. Trends Biochem Sci 1993;18:128–131.
21 Roulston A, Reinhard C, Amiri P, Williams LT: Early activation of c-Jun N-terminal kinase and p38 kinase regulate cell survival in response to tumor necrosis factor-α. J Biol Chem 1998;17:10232–10239.
22 Beyaert R, Kidd VJ, Cornelis S, Van de Craen M, Denecker G, Lahti JM, Gururajan R, Vandenabeele P, Fiers W: The p38/RK mitogen-activated protein kinase pathway regulates interleukin-6 synthesis response to tumor necrosis factor. EMBO J 1996;15:1914–1923.
23 Beg AA, Baltimore D: An essential role for NF-κB in preventing TNF-α-induced cell death. Science 1996;274:782–784.
24 Wang C-Y, Mayo MW, Baldwin AS Jr: TNF- and cancer therapy-induced apoptosis: Potentiation by inhibition of NF-κB. Science 1996; 274:784–787.
25 Antwerp DJV, Martin SJ, Kafri T, Green DR, Verma IM: Suppression of TNF-α-induced apoptosis by NF-κB. Science 1996;274:787–789.
26 Pazdrak K, Olszewska-Pazdrak B, Stafford S, Garofalo RP, Alam R: Lyn, Jak2, and Raf-1 kinases are critical for the antiapoptotic effect of interleukin-5, whereas only Raf-1 kinase is essential for eosinophil activation and degranulation. J Exp Med 1998;188:421–429.

International Archives of
Allergy and
Immunology

Int Arch Allergy Immunol 1999;120(suppl 1):60–64

Mechanisms of Eosinophil Cationic Protein Release in the Serum: Role of Adhesion Molecules

Yoshiko Kato[a] Takao Fujisawa[b] Akihiko Terada[b] Kosei Iguchi[b]
Hitoshi Kamiya[b]

[a]Department of Psychiatry, University of Mie School of Medicine, and [b]Department of Pediatrics, Mie National Hospital, Tsu, Mie, Japan

Key Words
Eosinophils · Eosinophil cationic protein · Serum · Adhesion molecules · Integrins

Abstract
Background: Measurement of eosinophil cationic protein (ECP) in serum has been utilized as a marker for allergic inflammation. The serum level of ECP represents the level found in vivo plus additional proteins released in vitro from peripheral blood eosinophils during the coagulation period. The mechanisms of release, however, are unclear. We investigated a possible involvement of adhesion molecules in the ECP release. ***Materials and Methods:*** Venous blood was drawn in the presence of EDTA from allergic donors. The blood was incubated with neutralizing monoclonal antibodies to CD18, CD11a, CD11b, CD29, CD49d, CD54, $\alpha_4\beta_7$, or isotype-matched control antibodies, respectively, at 4 °C for 30 min. Calcium gluconate (calcium) was then added to induce coagulation. The blood was further incubated for 90 min and centrifuged to obtain the serum. ECP in the serum was measured with RIA. In some experiments, purified eosinophils were incubated with plasma and calcium, then ECP in the supernatants was assayed. ***Results:*** ECP in the samples with calcium was significantly higher than in those without calcium. Purified eosinophils released ECP upon plasma coagulation. Anti-CD18, CD49d, and $\alpha_4\beta_7$ antibodies significantly suppressed ECP levels in the serum. ***Conclusions:*** These results suggest that ECP release in the serum is calcium and plasma coagulation-dependent and that cell adhesion through $\alpha_L\beta_2$, $\alpha_M\beta_2$, $\alpha_4\beta_1$ and $\alpha_4\beta_7$ integrins is at least in part responsible for ECP release.

Introduction

Eosinophil infiltration into the airway wall is one of the characteristic features of the pathology of bronchial asthma. Eosinophils play a central role in causing bronchial hyperresponsiveness through the damage of airway epithelium and are major effector cells in allergic inflammation. Various mediators contribute to effector function of eosinophils. Among them, cationic proteins of the specific granules have a high toxicity to normal tissue [1] and pleiotropic biologic activities related to pathogenesis of asthma [2]. Therefore measurement of eosinophil granule proteins, namely, eosinophil cationic protein (ECP) and major basic protein, in serum, sputum, and bronchoalveolar lavage fluid has been utilized as a marker for eosinophilic inflammation. Because of its easier accessibility,

KARGER

Fax + 41 61 306 12 34
E-Mail karger@karger.ch
www.karger.com

1018–2438/99/1205–0060$17.50/0

Accessible online at:
http://BioMedNet.com/karger

Takao Fujisawa, MD
Mie National Hospital
357 Osato-kubota
Tsu City, Mie 514-0125 (Japan)

ECP in the serum has been most widely studied and reported to have significant correlations with symptoms, pulmonary functions, bronchial hyperresponsiveness, and response to therapeutic interventions in asthma [3–5]. The serum level of ECP represents the level found in vivo plus additional proteins released in vitro from peripheral blood eosinophils during the coagulation period and is believed to express 'activation' status of peripheral blood eosinophils. Mechanisms of the release, however, are not well understood. To further understand the role of eosinophils in pathogenesis of allergic diseases, factors that induce ECP release in the serum have to be clarified. We hypothesized that the cell activation through adhesion molecules may be involved in the release of ECP in the serum.

Materials and Methods

The monoclonal antibodies (mAb) to CD18 (clone L130, mouse IgG1) and CD11b (clone D12, mouse IgG2a) were purchased from Becton Dickinson (San Jose, Calif., USA). Anti-CD11a (clone 25.3.1, mouse IgG1), anti-CD54 (clone 84H10, mouse IgG1), anti-CD49d (clone HP2/1, mouse IgG1), and anti-CD29 (clone Lia1/2, mouse IgG1) were from Immunotech (Marseille, France). Anti-$\alpha_4\beta_7$ (clone ACT-1, mouse IgG1) was a kind gift from Leukosite (Cambridge, Mass., USA). Irrelevant isotype-matched mAbs, mouse IgG1 and IgG2a were purchased from Zymed Laboratories (San Francisco, Calif., USA).

Venous blood was drawn from volunteers with asthma or atopic dermatitis and EDTA at 2.5 m*M* and mAbs at 20 µg/ml were promptly added to the blood. After incubation at 4°C for 30 min, calcium gluconate at 5 m*M* was added to the sample to induce coagulation. To simulate a standard blood processing method [4], the sample was allowed to clot at room temperature for 90 min, and then centrifuged at 1,000 *g* for 10 min to obtain the serum. The serum level of ECP was measured with a double-antibody RIA kit (Pharmacia Diagnostics, Uppsala, Sweden). In some experiments, eosinophils were purified with Percoll density centrifugation and a magnetic cell separation system (MACS®, Miltenyi Biotec, Germany) [6]. Plasma from the same donor containing heparin or EDTA was also separated. Plasma samples were processed to be platelet-rich or devoid of platelets by centrifuging the blood at 225 or 1,050 *g*, respectively. Purified eosinophils and each preparation of plasma were mixed and incubated at room temperature for 90 min upon addition of calcium. ECP in the supernatants was measured after centrifugation.

Data were expressed as mean ± SEM. Statistical analysis was performed by Mann-Whitney U test and Wilcoxon signed rank test.

Results and Discussion

The main objective of this study was to investigate whether adhesion molecules on eosinophils were involved in ECP release in the serum and we utilized antiadhesion molecule antibodies. Because ECP is known to be released during blood clotting, the antibodies have to be added before the clotting process. Therefore we divided the blood processing procedure for serum ECP measurement into two phases, the antibody incubation phase with EDTA and the coagulation phase with calcium gluconate. First, it was confirmed that calcium gluconate added at 5 m*M* completely reversed the anticoagulant effect of EDTA at 2.5 m*M*. After 90 min of incubation, ECP levels in the supernatant (serum) with calcium were significantly higher than without (fig. 1), suggesting that ECP release in the blood is calcium-dependent.

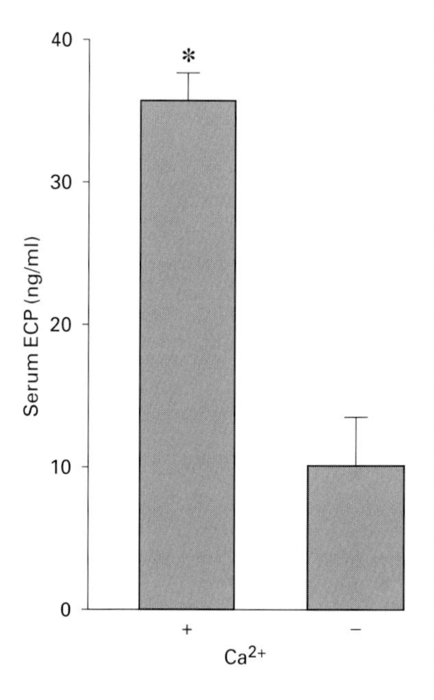

Fig. 1. Calcium-dependent release of ECP in the serum. Venous blood was drawn in the presence of EDTA from allergic donors. Calcium gluconate at 5 m*M* was added to the blood to induce coagulation. An equal volume of PBS was added as control. The blood was then incubated at room temperature for 90 min and centrifuged to obtain serum. ECP in the serum was measured with RIA. * $p < 0.05$ (n = 5).

Next, the effect of antiadhesion molecule antibodies was tested. Anti-CD18 and combinations of anti-CD18 (β_2 integrin) and CD11a (α_L integrin), CD18 and CD11b (α_M integrin), CD18 and CD54 (ICAM-1) significantly inhibited the ECP release (fig. 2). Anti-CD49d (α_4 integrin), a combination of anti-CD49d and CD29 (β_1 integrin) (fig. 3), and anti-$\alpha_4\beta_7$ (fig. 4) also suppressed the release. A single use of antibodies to CD11a, CD11b, and CD29 did not show a significant effect. These results sug-

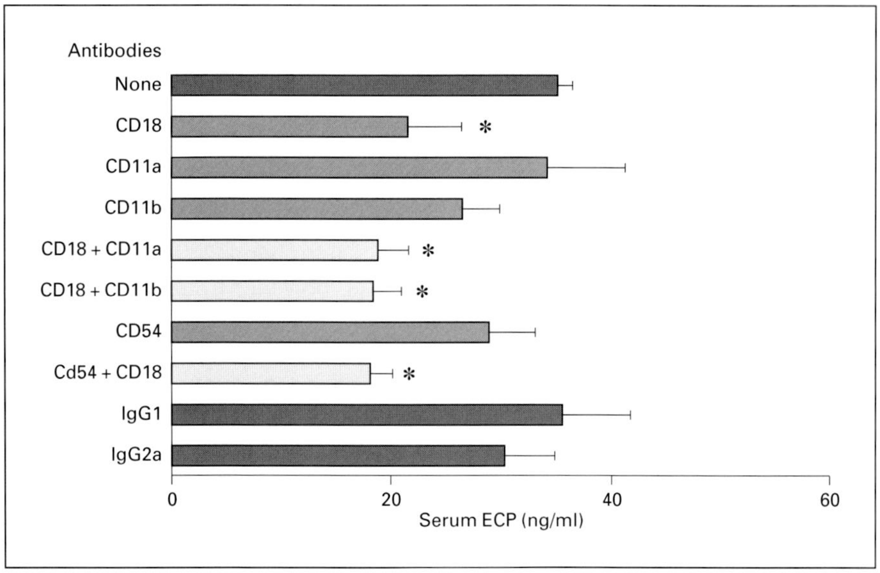

Fig. 2. Effect of antiadhesion molecule antibodies on serum ECP release (experiment 1). * $p < 0.05$ (n = 5).

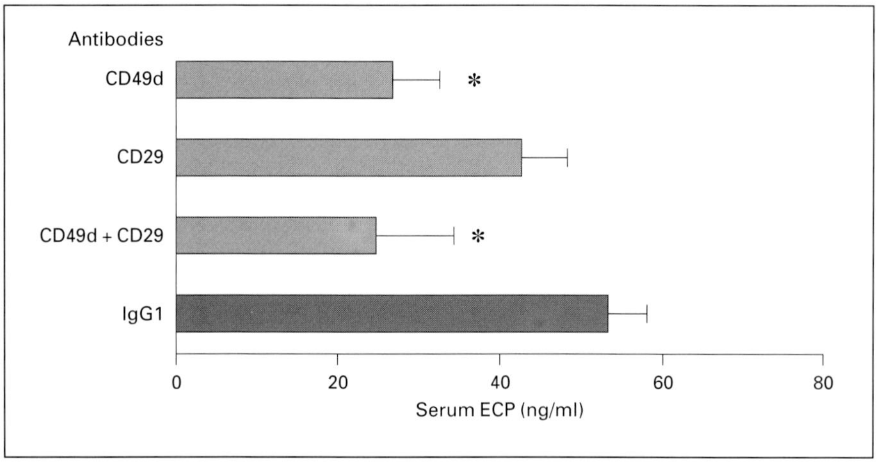

Fig. 3. Effect of antiadhesion molecule antibodies on serum ECP release (experiment 2). * $p < 0.05$ (n = 5).

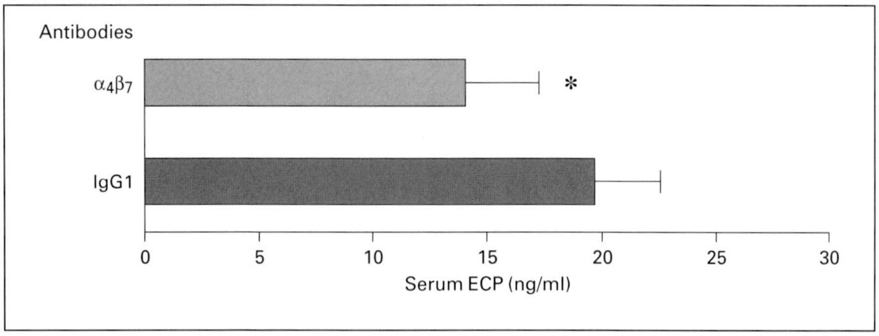

Fig. 4. Effect of antiadhesion molecule antibodies on serum ECP release (experiment 3). * $p < 0.05$ (n = 7).

gest that integrins $\alpha_L\beta_2$, $\alpha_M\beta_2$, $\alpha_4\beta_1$ and $\alpha_4\beta_7$ may be involved in the ECP release in the serum. It has been reported that β_2 integrins are necessary for effector functions of eosinophils such as IgG, PAF, IL-5 and GM-CSF-induced degranulation and superoxide generation [7–10]. In these experiments, eosinophils incubated with the stimulants adhering to the culture plate and anti-CD18 blocked the adhesion as well as degranulation. Protein tyrosine phosphorylation and phosphoinositide turnover were also observed upon stimulation [10], indicating that

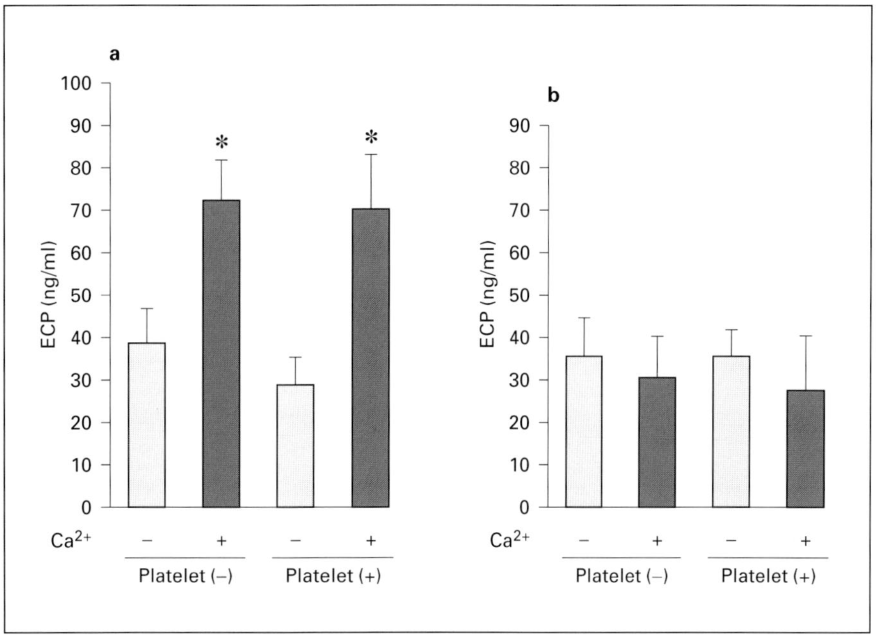

Fig. 5. ECP release and plasma coagulation. Purified eosinophils were incubated with the plasma that was processed with EDTA (**a**) or heparin (**b**) from the same donor. The plasma was either platelet-rich or devoid of platelets, which was obtained by centrifuging blood to which EDTA or heparin had been added at 225 *g* to include platelets, or at 1,050 *g* to remove them. Then calcium gluconate was added. After 90 min of incubation, the samples were centrifuged and ECP in the supernatants was measured with RIA. * $p < 0.05$ (n = 6).

cellular adhesion through β_2 integrin triggers activation of an intracellular signaling, which is then followed by eosinophil effector functions. Cellular adhesion through β_1 integrins has also been reported to trigger eosinophil functions [11]. In this study, we found that ECP release in the serum required the involvement of the integrins. The serum levels of ECP have been reported to be elevated in patients with various allergic diseases [5, 12, 13]. The expression or activation state of the integrins may be enhanced in these patients and may be related to the elevated levels of serum ECP.

The ligands for the integrins in this system, however, are yet to be determined. Lymphocytes expressing ICAM-1 may be possible candidates since enhanced expression of ICAM-1 on peripheral blood CD4+ and CD8+ T cells from patients with a dual asthmatic reaction by allergen challenge has been reported [14]. Plasma proteins such as fibrinogen and fibronectin, which can bind to $\alpha_M\beta_2$, $\alpha_4\beta_1$ and $\alpha_4\beta_7$ integrins, are other possible candidates. We then tested the effect of plasma in this study. Coagulation was not observed in the plasma with heparin and calcium. Purified eosinophils incubated with heparin plasma did not release further ECP when calcium was added (fig. 5b). On the contrary, plasma with EDTA clotted upon addition of calcium and ECP levels were significantly higher in the samples with calcium than in those without (fig. 5a). The presence of platelets did not affect the release. These results suggested that plasma coagulation, not platelets, was required for the ECP release. Although molecular changes of plasma protein during coagulation and the plasma protein involved in the ECP release are not known in this system, it is possible that the quantitation of the protein in combination with ECP may be utilized as a marker for allergic inflammation. Further studies to clarify detailed mechanisms of serum ECP release have to be done.

References

1 Motojima S, Frigas E, Loegering DA, Gleich GJ: Toxicity of eosinophil cationic proteins for guinea pig tracheal epithelium in vitro. Am Rev Respir Dis 1989;139:801–805.

2 Gleich GJ, Adolphson CR, Leiferman KM: The biology of the eosinophilic leukocyte. Annu Rev Med 1993;44:85–101.

3 Zimmerman B, Lanner A, Enander I, Zimmerman RS, Peterson CGB, Ahlstedt S: Total blood eosinophils, serum eosinophil cationic protein and eosinophil protein X in childhood asthma: Relation to disease status and therapy. Clin Exp Allergy 1993;23:564–570.

4 Venge P: Serum measurements of eosinophil cationic protein (ECP) in bronchial asthma. Clin Exp Allergy 1993;23(suppl 2):3–7.

5 Fujisawa T, Terada J, Atsuta J, Iguchi K, Kamiya H: Clinical utility of serum levels of eosinophil cationic protein (ECP) for monitoring and predicting clinical course in childhood asthma. Clin Exp Allergy 1998;28:19–25.

6 Atsuta J, Fujisawa T, Iguchi K, Terada A, Kamiya H, Sakurai M: Inhibitory effect of transforming growth factor b1 on cytokine-enhanced eosinophil survival and degranulation. Int Arch Allergy Immunol 1995;108 (suppl 1):31–35.

7 Horie S, Kita H: CD11b/CD18 (Mac-1) is required for degranulation of human eosinophils induced by human recombinant granulocyte-macrophage colony-stimulating factor and platelet-activating factor. J Immunol 1994;152: 5457–5467.

8 Kaneko M, Horie S, Kato M, Gleich GJ, Kita H: A crucial role for β_2 integrin in the activation of eosinophils stimulated by IgG. J Immunol 1995;155:2631–2641.

9 Fujisawa T, Terada A, Atsuta J, Iguchi K, Kamiya H, Sakurai M: IL-5 as a strong secretagogue for human eosinophils. Int Arch Allergy Immunol 1997;114:81–83.

10 Kato M, Abraham RT, Okada S, Kita H: Ligation of the β2 integrin triggers activation and degranulation of human eosinophils. Am J Respir Cell Mol Biol 1998;18:675–686.

11 Nagata M, Sedgwick JB, Bates ME, Kita H, Busse WW: Eosinophil adhesion to vascular cell adhesion molecule-1 activates superoxide anion generation. J Immunol 1995;155:2194–2202.

12 Tomassini M, Magrini L, De Petrillo G, Adriani E, Bonini S, Balsano F: Serum levels of eosinophil cationic protein in allergic diseases and natural allergen exposure. J Allergy Clin Immunol 1996;97:1350–1355.

13 Halmerbauer G, Frischer T, Koller DY: Monitoring of disease activity by measurement of inflammatory markers in atopic dermatitis in childhood. Allergy 1997;52:765–769.

14 De Rose V, Rolla G, Bucca C, et al: Intercellular adhesion molecule-1 is upregulated on peripheral blood T lymphocyte subsets in dual asthmatic responders. J Clin Invest 1994;94: 1840–1845.

International Archives of
Allergy and Immunology

Int Arch Allergy Immunol 1999;120(suppl 1):65–69

Matrix Metalloproteinase-9 in Peripheral Blood Eosinophils

Takao Fujisawa[a] Yoshiko Kato[b] Akihiko Terada[a] Kosei Iguchi[a]
Hitoshi Kamiya[a]

[a]Department of Pediatrics, Mie National Hospital, and [b]Department of Psychiatry, University of Mie School of Medicine, Tsu, Mie, Japan

Key Words
Eosinophils · Matrix metalloproteinase-9 · Neutrophils · IL-5 · Phorbol myristate acetate

Abstract
Background: Matrix metalloproteinases (MMPs) are major contributors to tumor invasion, remodeling of connective tissue and infiltration of inflammatory cells and may be important mediators in developing allergic inflammation. Overexpression of MMP-9 mRNA by eosinophils in the asthmatic airways has been reported. To clarify the relative significance of MMP as an inflammatory mediator from eosinophils, we determined the content of MMP-9 in the peripheral blood eosinophils and compared it with the other leukocyte fractions. ***Methods:*** Peripheral blood eosinophils, neutrophils, and mononuclear cells were purified from normal and allergic donors with Percoll gradient centrifugation and CD16 negative selection. Cell lysate and culture supernatants stimulated with IL-5, PAF, and PMA were tested for MMP-9 with gelatin zymography and ELISA. ***Results:*** The amount of MMP-9 in highly purified eosinophils, neutrophils, and mononuclear cells was 2.5 ± 0.9, 4,073 ± 581, and 7.6 ± 1.4 ng/5 × 10^6 cells, respectively. There was no difference in MMP-9 content of eosinophils between normal donors and patients with asthma. Culture of peripheral blood eosinophils with IL-5 for 4 days did not induce MMP-9 production. The stimulation of eosinophils with PMA and other secretogogues caused only small amounts of MMP-9 secretion as compared with neutrophils. ***Conclusions:*** These findings suggest that circulating eosinophils normally have only small amounts of MMP-9 and that eosinophils may need complex activation signals to produce significant amounts of MMP as seen in tissues of allergic inflammation.

Introduction

Matrix metalloproteinases (MMPs) are a family of related zinc-containing enzymes capable of hydrolyzing tissue matrix components and have been implicated in connective tissue destruction in rheumatoid arthritis, tumor invasion, and inflammatory cell infiltration in certain inflammatory disorders [1, 2]. However, the role of MMPs in developing chronic inflammation and remodeling in allergic diseases is yet to be defined. Overexpression of MMP-9, or gelatinase B, by eosinophils in lung tissue from patients with asthma has been documented [3]. Elevated levels of MMP-9 in bronchoalveolar lavage fluid

KARGER
Fax + 41 61 306 12 34
E-Mail karger@karger.ch
www.karger.com

1018–2438/99/1205–0065$17.50/0

Accessible online at:
http://BioMedNet.com/karger

Takao Fujisawa, MD
Mie National Hospital
357 Osato-kubota
Tsu City, Mie 514-0125 (Japan)

from untreated asthmatics, in which alveolar macrophages were implied to be the source of the protease, have also been reported [4]. Here, we investigated whether the eosinophil, a major effector cell in allergic inflammation, is an important source of MMP-9 by quantitative analysis of the enzyme stored and released from eosinophils.

Materials and Methods

Human recombinant IL-5 was a kind gift from Suntory Institute of Biochemical Research (Osaka, Japan). Phorbol 12-myristate 13-acetate (PMA) and platelet-activating factor (PAF) were purchased from Sigma Chemical Co. (St. Louis, Mo., USA).

Eosinophils, neutrophils, and mononuclear cells were isolated from peripheral blood of normal and atopic donors with asthma or mild allergic rhinitis by the method described below. Briefly, leukocyte-rich plasma obtained by dextran sedimentation of heparinized peripheral blood were loaded on Percoll discontinuous density gradients (1.07, 1.08, 1.085, 1.09, 1.095) and centrifuged at 1,500 *g* for 10 min. Cell fractions at densities of around 1.07 and 1.08 were collected as mononuclear cells (fraction M) and neutrophils (fraction N), respectively. Eosinophils were further purified from fractions with densities over 1.085 by incubation with anti-CD16 antibody-coated MACS(r) beads (Miltenyi Biotec, Germany), followed by a negative selection step with a magnetic column to eliminate contaminating neutrophils (fraction E) [5]. The cell differential of each fraction was then determined by enumerating 500 cells in Giemsa-stained cytocentrifuge preparations. To ensure that detected MMP-9 was solely from eosinophils, samples of fraction E that were not of an eosinophil purity of 100% were excluded from the study. Fraction E was resuspended at 5×10^6 cells/ml, and fractions M and N were at 2.5×10^6 cells/ml in serum-free HybriCare medium (American Type Culture Collection, Rockville, Md., USA) with 0.1% human serum albumin (Sigma). One hundred microliters of cell suspension and 100 µl of PMA or IL-5 were incubated in 6-ml round-bottom culture tubes (Falcon; Becton-Dickinson, Lincoln Park, N.J., USA), at 37 °C for the indicated periods. Cell lysates with 5% Triton X-100, supernatants of cultured eosinophils and neutrophils with PMA, IL-5, and/or PAF were subjected to MMP assays.

MMPs were detected by gelatin zymography as described elsewhere [6]. Briefly, samples were diluted into a buffer consisting of 126 m*M* Tris-HCl, pH 6.8, 20% glycerol, 4% SDS, 0.005% bromophenol blue, then electrophoresed for 1.5 h at 4 °C on a precast 10% polyacrylamide minigel containing 0.1% gelatin (TEFCO, Tokyo, Japan) in a running buffer consisting of 25 m*M* Tris, 192 m*M* glycine, and 0.1% SDS. The gel was then incubated for 30 min at room temperature in renaturing buffer consisting of 2.5% Triton X-100 and 1 µ*M* $ZnCl_2$ on a rotary shaker. The gel was further incubated at 37 °C for 24 h with a buffer consisting of 10 m*M* Tris base, 40 m*M* Tris HCl, 200 m*M* NaCl, 10 m*M* $CaCl_2$, and 1 µ*M* $ZnCl_2$. The gel was stained with 0.5% Coomassie blue R-250 in 30% methanol, 10% acetic acid for 3 h and then destained with three changes of 30% methanol and 10% acetic acid. Areas of digestion were visualized as nonstaining regions of the gel. Quantitation of MMP-9 was performed with a specific ELISA kit (Amersham, UK), which detects the proform of MMP-9 and proMMP-9/TIMP-1 complex.

Table 1. Cell differentials of fractions of peripheral blood leukocytes separated by Percoll density gradient centrifugation and CD16 negative selection

Fraction	Cell differentials	Percentage
E	eosinophils	100
N	neutrophils	96.8±0.9
	eosinophils	3.1±1.0
M	lymphocytes	72.5±4.6
	monocytes	28.3±5.2
	basophils	0.2±0.1
	neutrophils	0.5±0.3
	eosinophils	0.04±0.04

Data are expressed as mean ± SEM of 5 donors.

Table 2. Changes in the content of MMP-9 in eosinophils cultured with IL-5

Culture, day	MMP-9, ng/5 × 10^6 cells
0	1.31±0.63
2	1.08±0.30
4	1.26±0.12

Purified eosinophils from mild atopic donors were cultured in the presence of IL-5 at 1 ng/ml and the cells were lysed with NP-40. Data were expressed as means ± SEM from 4 experiments of different donors.

Results and Discussion

Three gelatinolytic activities were detected in samples from eosinophil lysates by zymography. Most of the abundant gelatinolytic activity was observed in the 92-kD area, which corresponds to the proform of MMP-9. Because MMP-9 represents the major MMP in eosinophils as previously reported [7], it was then quantified using ELISA, and the content was compared among three different fractions of peripheral blood leukocytes. The amount of MMP-9 in fractions E, N, and M from normal or mildly atopic patients was 2.5 ± 0.9, 4,073 ± 581, and 7.6 ± 1.4 ng/5 × 10^6 cells, respectively (fig. 1). Cell differentials of the fractions are shown in table 1. Fraction E solely included eosinophils and fraction N mostly neutrophils with little contamination of eosinophils. Fraction M

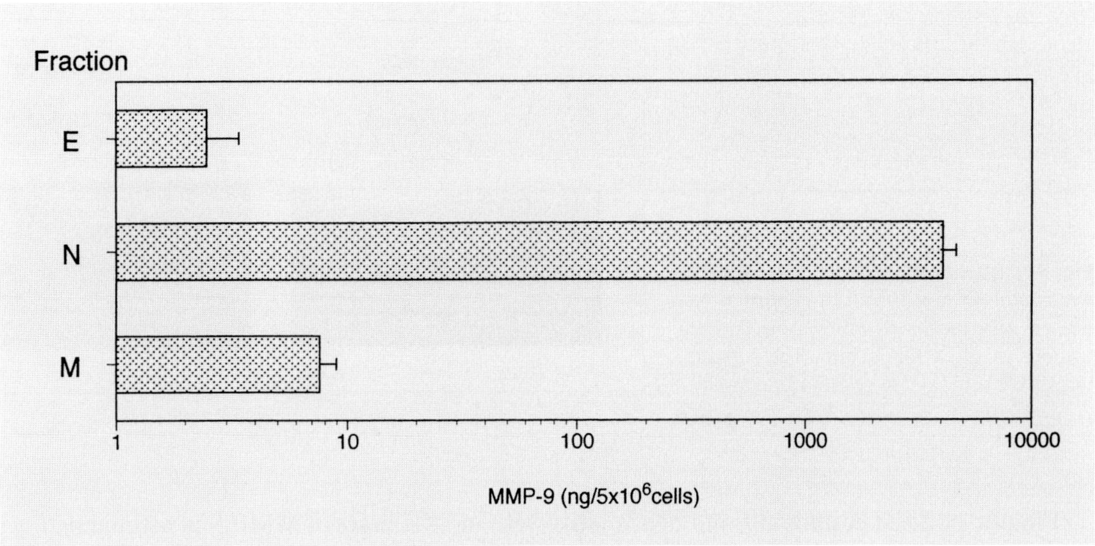

Fig. 1. Stored MMP-9 in different leukocyte fractions from peripheral blood. The cells were separated by the procedure described in Materials and Methods and lysed with 5% Triton X-100. The lysate of 5 × 10^6 cells was assayed for MMP-9 by ELISA. The data were expressed as means ± SEM of 5 donors.

mostly consisted of lymphocytes and monocytes. These results reveal that eosinophils and mononuclear cells contain significantly less MMP-9 than neutrophils.

Because of the previously reported abundant expression of MMP-9 mRNA by eosinophils in bronchial tissues of asthmatics [3], we then measured MMP-9 in eosinophils from patients with asthma. There was, however, no difference in the levels of stored MMP-9 between controls and patients with asthma (fig. 2). We further tested whether long-term culture with IL-5 may induce a higher expression of MMP-9 in eosinophils. Purified eosinophils from 4 atopic donors were cultured with IL-5 at 1 ng/ml for 4 days, and total cell lysates were assayed for MMP-9 with ELISA. The content of MMP-9 was not enhanced by IL-5 (table 2). Viability of the cells at 4 days of culture was 97.7 ± 0.8%. These results suggest that in terms of MMP-9, the phenotype of peripheral blood eosinophils is different from that of tissue eosinophils that have an enhanced expression of the protease, if any. However, we observed time-dependent increase of gelatinolytic activity at 92 kD in cultured eosinophils with IL-5 in a patient with severe atopic dermatitis. In this patient, quantification of the supernatant at 96 h revealed an MMP-9 level of 2.6 ng/1.7 × 10^6 cells, or 7.6 ng/5 × 10^6 cells. The MMP-9 level of 0 h lysate at 1.7 × 10^6 cells/ml was below the detection limit of 0.6 ng/ml by ELISA. Although this is an anecdotal observation, it is still possible that MMP-9 may be induced in peripheral blood eosinophils.

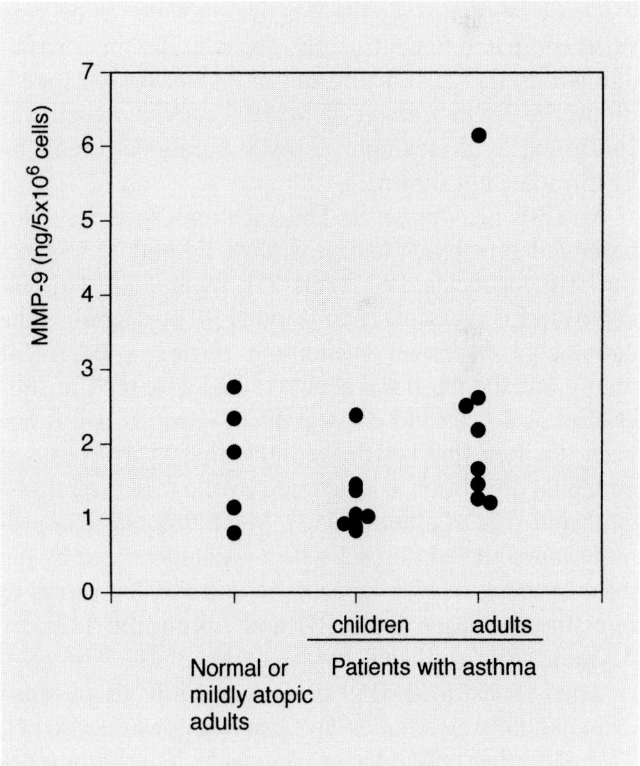

Fig. 2. MMP-9 content of freshly isolated eosinophils from normal and asthmatic donors. Eosinophils were separated by the procedure described in Materials and Methods and lysed with 5% Triton X-100. The lysate of 5 × 10^6 cells was assayed for MMP-9 by ELISA.

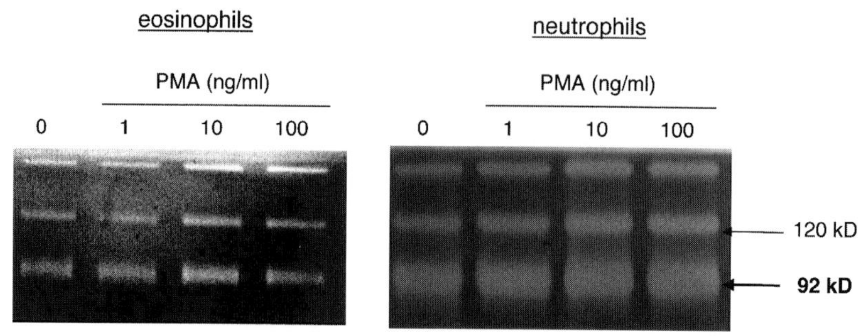

Fig. 3. Purified eosinophils at 3 × 10^6/ml or neutrophils at 1 × 10^6/ml from normal volunteers were incubated with various concentrations of PMA for 30 min. The supernatants were subjected to gelatin zymography.

Finally, purified eosinophils and neutrophils were incubated with PMA at 10 ng/ml for 30 min and supernatants were tested for MMPs. Major gelatinolytic activity in the culture supernatants of both cell types was in the 92 kD (fig. 3). The released MMP-9 in the supernatants was 1.1 ± 0.5 ng/5 × 10^6 cells for eosinophils and 1,321 ± 316 ng/5 × 10^6 cells for neutrophils (n = 5). The MMP-9 release from eosinophils was again shown to be very small compared to neutrophils. The stimulation of eosinophils with IL-5 at 10 ng/ml and/or PAF at 10^{-7} *M* for 2 h induced a small amount of MMP-9 release, which was confirmed by zymography and was barely detectable by ELISA (data not shown).

MMP-9 (gelatinase B) has substrate specificity for basement membrane collagens, type IV and V, connective-tissue-associated collagens VII, IX and XI. This enzyme increases vascular permeability [8] by degrading the endothelial basement membrane. Using a basement membrane model, it was shown to facilitate the transmigration of T cells and eosinophils in vitro [9, 10]. It has been reported that gelatinases including MMP-9 caused epithelial disruption as evidenced by the increased transepithelial flux of albumin [11]. MMP-9 could also promote subepithelial fibrosis, which is characterized by the disappearance of type IV collagen and the deposition of interstitial collagen (type III) and fibronectin [12], by degrading the epithelial basement membrane. In vivo, elevated levels of MMP-9 protein and mRNA in bronchial tissues of asthmatics have been demonstrated [3, 4]. Taken together, MMP-9 may contribute to the pathogenesis of asthma, which is characterized by mucosal edema, eosinophil and T cell accumulation, epithelial damage and remodeling.

Eosinophils [3], alveolar macrophages [4], and bronchial epithelium [11] have been implicated to be the sources of MMP-9 in asthma pathogenesis. As eosinophil is a major effector cell in allergic inflammation, we examined eosinophils as the possible source of MMP-9. Freshly isolated peripheral blood eosinophils, however, stored and released very small amounts of MMP-9, even in patients with asthma. Although this suggests that the eosinophil is a poor source, small amounts of the protease may be sufficient to cause eosinophils in close contact transmigrate through the basement membrane [10]. In addition, as our preliminary data have shown that cultured eosinophils with IL-5 produced larger amounts of MMP-9 than fresh counterparts, eosinophil-activating cytokines may trigger eosinophils to synthesize the protease as they infiltrate from the peripheral blood to the target tissue. Further studies will be required to clarify the source and pathophysiologic role of MMPs in bronchial asthma.

References

1 Stetler-Stevenson WG: Dynamics of matrix turnover during pathologic remodeling of the extracellular matrix. Am J Pathol 1996;148: 1345–1350.

2 Liotta LA, Stetler-Stevenson WG: Metalloproteinases and cancer invasion. Cancer Biol 1990;1:99–106.

3 Ohno I, Ohtani H, Nitta Y, Suzuki J, Hoshi H, Honma M, Isoyama S, Tanno Y, Tamura G, Yamauchi K, Nagura H, Shirato K: Eosinophils as a source of matrix metalloproteinase-9 in asthmatic airway inflammation. Am J Respir Cell Mol Biol 1997;16:212–219.

4 Mautino G, Oliver N, Chanez P, Bousquet J, Capony F: Increased release of matrix metalloproteinase-9 in bronchoalveolar lavage fluid and by alveolar macrophages of asthmatics. Am J Respir Cell Mol Biol 1997;17:583–591.

5 Atsuta J, Fujisawa T, Iguchi K, Terada A, Kamiya H, Sakurai M: Inhibitory effect of transforming growth factor beta1 on cytokine-enhanced eosinophil survival and degranulation. Int Arch Allergy Immunol 1995; 108(suppl 1):31–35.

6 Romanic AM, Madri JA: The induction of 72-kD gelatinase in T cells upon adhesion to endothelial cells is VCAM-1 dependent. J Cell Biol 1994;125:1165–1178.

7 Stahle-Backdahl M, Inoue M, Giudice GJ, Parks WC: 92-kD gelatinase is produced by eosinophils at the site of blister formation in bullous pemphigoid and cleaves the extracellular domain of recombinant 180-kD bullous pemphigoid autoantigen. J Clin Invest 1994; 93:2022–2030.

8 Partridge CA, Jeffrey JJ, Malik AB: A 96-kDa gelatinase induced by TNF-alpha contributes to increased microvascular endothelial permeability. Am J Physiol 1993;265:438–447.

9 Leppert D, Waubant E, Galardy R, Bunnett NW, Hauser SL: T cell gelatinases mediate basement membrane transmigration in vitro. J Immunol 1995;154:4379–4389.

10 Okada S, Kita H, George TJ, Gleich GJ, Leiferman KM: Migration of eosinophils through basement membrane components in vitro: Role of matrix metalloproteinase-9. Am J Respir Cell Mol Biol 1997;17:519–528.

11 Herbert CA, Arthur MJP, Robinson C: Augmentation by eosinophils of gelatinase activity in the airway mucosa: Comparative effects as a putative mediator of eosinophil injury. Br J Clin Pharmacol 1996;117:667–674.

12 Roche WR, Beasley R, Williams J, Holgate ST: Subepithelial fibrosis in the bronchi of asthmatics. Lancet 1989;8637:520–524.

International Archives of
Allergy and Immunology

Int Arch Allergy Immunol 1999;120(suppl 1):70–75

NC/Nga Mice: A Mouse Model for Atopic Dermatitis

Hajime Suto[a,b] Hiroshi Matsuda[c] Koichi Mitsuishi[a,b] Kayako Hira[a,b] Takafumi Uchida[a,b,d] Tetsushi Unno[a,b] Hideoki Ogawa[a,b] Chisei Ra[a,d]

[a]Atopy and Allergy Research Center, and [b]Department of Dermatology, Juntendo University School of Medicine, Tokyo, [c]Department of Veterinary Clinic, Faculty of Agriculture, Tokyo University of Agriculture and Technology, and [d]Department of Immunology, Juntendo University School of Medicine, Tokyo, Japan

Key Words

Atopic dermatitis · NC/Nga mouse · Mouse model · IgE · Mast cell · Eosinophil

Abstract

Atopic dermatitis (AD) is a common pruritic disease that occurs primarily in infancy and childhood. AD is characterized by itching and the patient having an individual or family history of atopic diseases. Although AD is also frequently associated with elevated serum IgE levels and with common environmental factors contributing to its pathogenesis, the etiology of AD is still unknown. We examined NC/Nga mice (NC mice) that showed AD-like skin lesions with aging as a possible mouse model for AD. NC mice were maintained under conventional (Conv) or specific pathogen-free (SPF) conditions. Clinical symptoms, serum IgE levels and histopathology of the skin were compared between these 2 groups, and we explored their application as a model of human AD. It was found that the skin lesions of inbred NC mice were clinically and histologically very similar to human AD when the mice were raised under Conv conditions, but not under SPF conditions, and we assumed that some kinds of environmental factors might trigger AD-like signs and symptoms in NC mice. To further investigate the pathophysiology and treatment of AD, a suitable animal model is absolutely required, and NC mice are very useful for this purpose.

Introduction

Atopic dermatitis (AD) is an itchy, chronic, or chronically relapsing, pruritic inflammatory skin disease. The patient usually has a family history of atopy [1, 2] which is obtained in about 70% of all cases. AD is frequently associated with elevated serum levels of IgE antibody against many kinds of inhaled, food and environmental allergens. About 80% of AD patients have increased amounts of total IgE [3]. Although the precise pathogenic mechanisms of AD are as yet unknown, evidence suggests that immunological abnormalities, such as type I and type IV allergy [3], barrier dysfunction [4–7], environmental factors and psychotic factors, contribute to the development and pathogenesis of AD. To further explore the pathophysiology and treatment of AD, a suitable animal model is required. Further study of the clinical symptoms, serum IgE levels and the histopathology of NC/Nga mice (NC mice) [8] has revealed their usefulness as a model for human AD.

KARGER

Fax + 41 61 306 12 34
E-Mail karger@karger.ch
www.karger.com

1018–2438/99/1205–0070$17.50/0

Accessible online at:
http://BioMedNet.com/karger

Chisei Ra, MD, PhD
Atopy and Allergy Research Center, Juntendo University School of Medicine
2-1-1 Hongo, Bunkyo-ku, Tokyo 113-8421 (Japan)
Tel. +81 3 3813 3111 (ext. 3546), Fax +81 3 3813 2205
E-Mail cra@med.juntendo.ac.jp

Materials and Methods

Mice

BALB/c mice were purchased from Nihon SLC (Shizuoka, Japan). NC mice were bred and housed at Tokyo University of Agriculture and Technology.

Clinical Examinations

Comparison of AD clinical scores of NC mice maintained under specific pathogen-free (SPF) and conventional (Conv) conditions was performed. Conv NC mice were maintained in ambient laboratory conditions in which air circulated without filtration. SPF NC mice were maintained in air-regulated conditions in which 99.7% of dust was removed from the circulated air with HEPA filters (mesh size: 0.3 µm; Clea, Tokyo, Japan). All other conditions were the same: temperature 23 ± 1.5 °C, relative humidity 60 ± 10%, and lighting 12 h on/12 h off. Both groups of mice were provided with γ-irradiated food and autoclaved water ad libitum.

We estimated the clinical severity of lesions in NC mice using the scores of Leung [9] and compared them between SPF NC mice and Conv NC mice. The total score for AD-like skin lesions was designated as the sum of individual scores graded as 0 (none), 1 (mild), 2 (moderate) and 3 (severe) for the symptoms of itch, erythema/hemorrhage, edema, excoriation/erosion and scaling/dryness.

Laboratory Examinations

Comparison of Consecutive Changes in Total Serum IgE Levels of NC Mice Maintained under SPF and Conv Conditions. We compared eosinophil counts of peripheral blood and total serum IgE levels between SPF NC and Conv NC mice. Blood was collected from the retro-orbital plexus under ether anesthesia and heparinized immediately thereafter. Plasma samples were obtained by centrifugation and stored at −20 °C until use. Total IgE levels were measured by sandwich ELISA using two kinds of rat anti-mouse IgE monoclonal antibodies (6HD5 and HMK 12) according to a method described previously [10]. Congo red staining was used for determination of eosinophils [11].

Histopathology of the Skin. (1) Comparison of the histopathology of skin lesions in NC mice maintained under SPF and Conv conditions. We compared the histopathological changes of the skin between SPF and Conv NC mice. Samples were obtained from dorsal skin before and after onset of the clinical symptoms and stained with hematoxylin-eosin (HE) and toluidine blue (TB). Small pieces of the samples were fixed in 10% phosphate-buffered formalin (pH 7.2), embedded in paraffin, cut at 4 µm, and stained with acidic TB (pH 4.0) for counting mast cells [12] and Congo red staining for counting eosinophils [11]. (2) Comparison of mast cell and eosinophil counts in the lesional skin of NC mice maintained under SPF and Conv conditions. We compared mast cell and eosinophil counts in the lesional skin of NC mice between SPF and Conv NC mice at 7 weeks of age (before onset of AD symptoms) and 17 weeks of age (after onset of AD symptoms) under a light microscope. Mast cells and eosinophils were counted under a microscope [13] at a magnification of × 400 and expressed as the total number of the cells in five fields. Each value was obtained from 7 mice per group. We also examined BALB/c mice as normal controls maintained with Conv NC mice under the same conditions in all experiments.

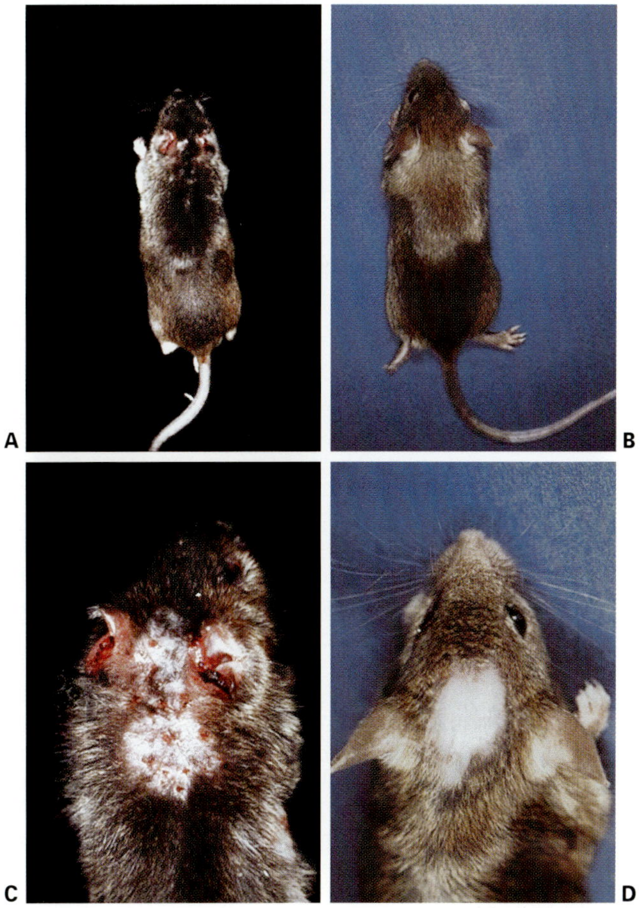

Fig. 1. Comparison of skin manifestations in NC mice maintained under SPF and Conv conditions at 24 weeks of age. **A** Conv NC mice (low-power view). **B** SPF NC mice (low-power view). **C** Conv NC mice (high-power view). **D** SPF NC mice (high-power view). On the ears, face, nose and dorsal skin, erythema, hemorrhage, excoriation, erosion, scaling and dryness were observed in Conv NC mice. No skin lesions were clinically detected in SPF NC mice.

Results

NC mice developed AD-like skin lesions when maintained under Conv but not under SPF conditions. It may be due to the severe itchiness and stresses that Conv NC mice with AD-like skin lesions appeared smaller (like suffering from growth retardation) than SPF NC mice of the same age. The hair of Conv NC mice was rougher than that of SPF NC mice, especially on the head and dorsal skin (fig. 1A). On the ears, face, nose, dorsal skin and almost everywhere, erythema, hemorrhage, excoriation, erosion, scaling and dryness were observed in Conv NC mice (fig. 1C). The signs began with scratching behavior and dry skin; erythema, eczematous lesions, and crusts of

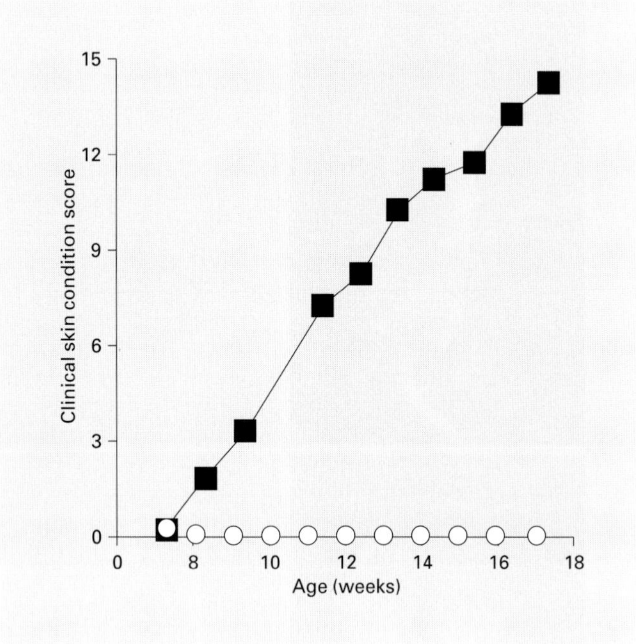

Fig. 2. Comparison of clinical skin condition scores of NC mice maintained under SPF and Conv conditions (n = 7). AD-like skin lesions could be detected from 8 weeks of age. Skin severity scores increased with age and reached more than 13 out of 15 points in mice 17 weeks of age under Conv conditions. In SPF NC and control BALB/c mice, the scores did not increase. ■ = Conv NC mice; ○ = SPF NC mice.

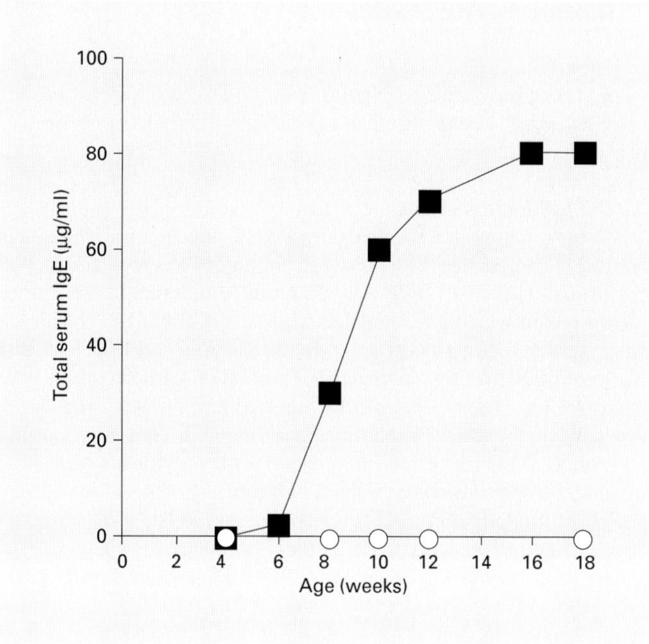

Fig. 3. Comparison of consecutive changes in total serum IgE levels (μg/ml) of NC mice maintained under SPF and Conv conditions (n = 7). Serum IgE levels of Conv NC mice increased from 6 weeks of age and reached a very high level (80 μg/ml). Serum IgE levels of SPF NC and control BALB/c mice remained at low levels of less than 0.5 μg/ml. ■ = Conv NC mice; ○ = SPF NC mice.

the skin developed gradually with aging in Conv NC mice. Even when Conv NC mice appeared normal at first inspection, eczema and crusts were seen under the hair. On the other hand, no skin lesions were clinically detected in SPF NC mice (fig. 1B). Even with high-power view, no eczematous lesions could be observed on the head skin of SPF NC mice (fig. 1D). BALB/c mice as controls, which were maintained with Conv NC mice under the same conditions, displayed no eczematous lesions like SPF NC mice.

To compare the skin lesions of NC mice, we utilized the clinical severity scores which were proposed by Leung [9] for human AD. AD-like skin lesions could be detected from 8 weeks of age, and the skin severity scores increased with age and reached more than 13 out of 15 points in 17-week-old mice under Conv conditions. On the other hand, SPF NC mice did not appear to have skin lesions (clinical severity score: 0 points) at over 32 weeks of age (fig. 2). Control BALB/c mice were maintained under the same conventional conditions with Conv NC mice, in the same cage, but the clinical severity scores of the control BALB/c mice stayed at 0 points as in SPF NC mice during the course of the experiments.

Serum IgE levels of the Conv NC mice increased from 6 weeks of age and reached very high levels (25 μg/ml) at 8 weeks of age, when mild dermatitis was clinically evident. The serum IgE levels in Conv NC mice correlated well with the clinical severity of AD, continued to increase to 70 μg/ml at 10 weeks and reached plateau at 17 weeks (300 μg/ml). In contrast, the serum IgE levels in SPF NC and control BALB/c mice remained at low levels of less than 0.5 μg/ml (fig. 3).

Histopathological examination was performed with HE staining of the involved skin (dorsal skin) in Conv and SPF NC mice. Although in Conv NC mice only minimal clinical signs or symptoms were observed at 7 weeks of age, there were already significant histopathological changes, such as infiltration of numerous eosinophils and a small number of mononuclear cells. Slight intercellular edema was present, but vesicle formation was not observed. Drastic changes in histopathology were noted at 17 weeks of age in Conv NC mice with severe skin lesions

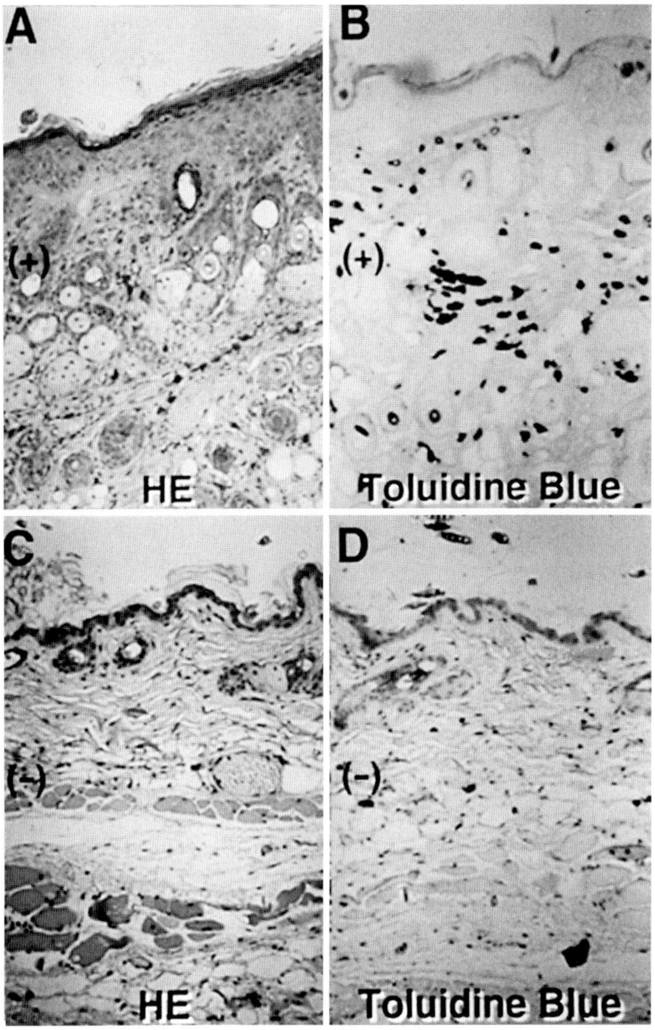

Fig. 4. Comparison of the histopathology of dorsal skin lesions in NC mice maintained under SPF and Conv conditions (17 weeks of age). **A** Conv NC mice. **B** Conv NC mice. **C** SPF NC mice. **D** SPF NC mice. Hyperkeratosis, acanthosis, exocytosis and moderate infiltration of mononuclear cells were revealed at 17 weeks of age. An increased number of mast cells with mild degranulation could be observed. SPF NC mice did not appear to have any eczematous changes.

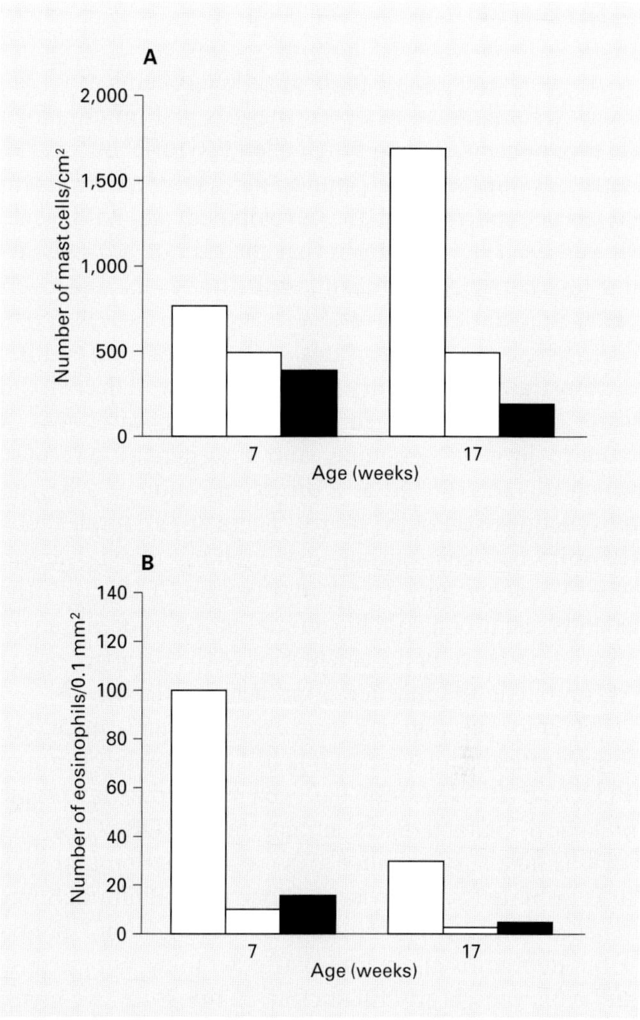

Fig. 5. Comparison of mast cell and eosinophil counts in the lesional skin of NC mice maintained under SPF and Conv conditions (Conv and SPF NC mice: n = 10; BALB/c mice: n = 5; mean ± SE). **A** Number of mast cells/cm^2. ▨ = Conv NC mice; □ = SPF NC mice; ■ = BALB/c mice. See Results for interpretation. **B** Number of eosinophils/0.1 mm^2. ▨ = Conv NC mice; □ = SPF NC mice; ■ = BALB/c mice. See Results for interpretation.

(fig. 4). Namely hyperkeratosis, acanthosis, exocytosis and moderate infiltration of mononuclear cells were revealed at that age. An increased number of mast cells with mild degranulation could also be observed (fig. 4).

Immunohistochemical examination of the skin lesions revealed increases in the numbers of mast cells and eosinophils (fig. 5). We observed an increase in mast cells at 7 weeks of age, and a remarkable increase could be detected at 17 weeks of age in Conv NC mice. Degranulation of activated mast cells was also observed (fig. 5A). No increase in mast cell counts was seen in control BALB/c and SPF NC mice (fig. 5A). In Conv NC mice, numerous eosinophils with slight or mild degranulation were observed in the involved skin at 7 weeks of age, and the eosinophil number was decreased to <301 at 17 weeks of age, although blood eosinophilia was still observed. The tissue eosinophils of SPF NC and control BALB/c mice remained within a normal range (fig. 5B) (<20/0.1 mm^2).

Discussion

Although the precise pathogenetic mechanisms of AD are as yet unknown, evidence suggests that immunological mechanisms, such as type I allergy, type IV allergy [3], barrier dysfunction [4–7], and some kinds of environmental factors, contribute to the development and pathogenesis of AD. It is well known that the skin of AD patients displays barrier dysfunction, tends to be dry and overreacts to irritation by a variety of antigens, viruses, fungi, even where water permeates the skin. Several studies demonstrated that the dry skin in AD shows a decrease in water content, enhanced transepidermal water loss, a reduced level of ceramide, and disorders of enzymes, which was interpreted as a direct reflection of a barrier dysfunction of the skin [14, 15]. There was a complex relationship between barrier dysfunction, type I allergy, type IV allergy and T cell dysfunction. Therefore, the establishment of a suitable animal model is definitely of great importance in the elucidation of the pathogenesis of AD and in developing new approaches to therapy [3].

NC mice [8] originate from Japanese fancy mice (Nishiki-Nezumi) and were established as an inbred strain in 1955. The NC/Nga strain has been reported to have some biological characteristics similar to the DBA/2 strain, such as high susceptibility to X-ray irradiation and high susceptibility to anaphylactic shock by ovalbumin. Some Japanese researchers noticed development of spontaneous dermatitis just before or after weaning, but its cause and pathogenesis are still unclear. In this study, we investigated whether the skin lesions which spontaneously develop in conventionally raised NC mice are comparable to human AD.

We compared the clinical features of NC mice maintained under SPF and Conv conditions. Only Conv NC mice, but not SPF NC mice, showed AD-like clinical symptoms with other atopic symptoms, such as allergic conjunctivitis (fig. 1C). Clinical symptoms began at 8 weeks of age with dryness of the skin and worsened continually until 17 weeks of age. Even when mice appeared normal without skin lesions, eczema and crusts were observed on the skin under the hair. On the other hand, no skin lesions were clinically detected in SPF NC mice (fig. 1B).

Next, we estimated the clinical scores of Conv NC mice and compared them with those of SPF NC and control BALB/c mice. Positive skin severity scores started at 8 weeks of age, increased with age and reached a maximum at 17 weeks of age. On the other hand, SPF NC and control BALB/c mice did not appear to have any clinical symptoms at over 32 weeks of age (fig. 2) and stayed at 0 points of the score. When several mating pairs of SPF NC mice were moved to a conventional room with uncontrolled air (Conv condition), various grades of dermatitis were clinically observed on the face, nose, neck, dorsal skin and everywhere, starting from the age of 8 weeks in all the progeny. In these experiments, SPF indicates only air-regulated circumstances, which means a laminar-filtered air flow enclosure in a biologically clean room. These results strongly suggest that the dermatitis observed in Conv NC mice was not simply due to a transmission of some kind of infectious agent, but due to some specific factors such as transepidermal, aerobic, and oral antigens.

The observation that IgE levels [16, 17] increased in association with clinical severity of dermatitis in Conv NC mice (fig. 3) was similar to that reported in AD patients with IgE hyperproduction. IgE synthesis in B cells is probably regulated by IL-4 that is produced by Th2-type helper T cells and by mast cells and basophils. We studied Th2-type cytokine (such as IL-4, IL-5 and IL-6) productivity of B cells of NC mice, which is actually accelerated in Conv NC mice (reported elsewhere). In the histopathological study of Conv NC mice, although only minimal clinical signs or symptoms were observed at 7 weeks of age, there were significant histopathological changes which developed with age. Drastic changes, such as hyperkeratosis, acanthosis, exocytosis and moderate infiltration of mononuclear cells were noted at 17 weeks of age in Conv NC mice with severe skin lesions (fig. 4).

The onset of dermatitis was histopathologically characterized by an increase in mast cells with mild degranulation and infiltration of numerous eosinophils at the skin lesion. Since a slight but significant elevation of serum total IgE levels was noted at 6 weeks, various kinds of chemical mediators and cytokines released from immunologically activated mast cells might lead to primary inflammation in the skin, including infiltration of eosinophils. Marked degranulation of eosinophils may release inflammatory factors, such as platelet-activating factor, leukotriene C4, RANTES, ECP (eosinophil cationic protein) and major basic protein (BMP) [3], which aggravates the condition of dermatitis [18]. In Conv NC mice, numerous eosinophils with slight or mild degranulation were observed in the involved skin at 7 weeks of age. At 17 weeks of age, eosinophil numbers were decreased to <30.1, and most of the remaining eosinophils were severely degranulated. Prominent eosinophilic material was deposited widely in the skin lesions shown by Congo red staining, suggesting that granule proteins such as MBP and ECP might be released from activated eosinophils in the skin lesions. Recently, we examined the barrier functions of the skin of NC mice and found a decrease in skin surface conductance, ceramide levels of stratum corneum and increased levels of transepidermal water loss. Those phenomena were found in Conv NC mice only, starting at 8 weeks of age. But on the other hand, SPF NC and BALB/c mice did not show such barrier dysfunctions and decreased levels of ceramide in stratum corneum at any time point (data not shown). Thus, these skin features and clinical symptoms of NC mice were similar to those in human AD.

In conclusion, clinical symptoms, laboratory data and histopathological findings in NC mice were very similar to those in human AD. The experiments described here suggest that NC mice are a suitable model for certain aspects of human AD and that their dermatitis with IgE hyperproduction is, at least in part, influenced by environmental factors.

References

1 Hanifin JM, Rajka G: Diagnostic features of atopic dermatitis. Acta Derm Venereol Suppl (Stockh) 1980;92:44–47.
2 Japanese Dermatological Association: Criteria for the Diagnosis of Atopic Dermatitis. J Dermatol 1995;22:966–967.
3 Leung DYM, Rhodes AR, Geha RS, Schneider L, Ring J: Atopic dermatitis (atopic eczema); in Fitzpatrick TB, Eisen AZ, Wolff K, Freedberg IM, Austen KF (eds): Dermatology in General Medicine, ed 4. New York, McGraw-Hill, 1993, pp 1543–1564.
4 Ogawa H: Fundamental pathogenesis of atopic dermatitis and that of alopecia areata. J Dermatol Sci 1990;1:375.
5 Ogawa H, Yoshiike T: A speculative view of atopic dermatitis. J Dermatol Sci 1993;5:197–204.
6 Yoshiike T, Aikawa Y, Sindhvananda J, Suto H, Nishimura K, Kawamoto T, Ogawa H: Skin barrier defect in atopic dermatitis: Increased permeability of the stratum corneum using dimethyl sulfoxide and theophylline. J Dermatol Sci 1993;5:92–96.
7 Aikawa Y, Yoshiike T: Studies of stratum corneum permeability in normal individuals and patients with atopic dermatitis utilizing a diffusion chamber system. Jpn J Dermatol 1997;107:1473–1478.
8 Matsuda H, Watanabe N, Geba GP, Sperl J, Tsudzuki M, Hiroi J, Matsumoto M, Ushio H, Saito S, Askenase PW, Ra C: Development of atopic dermatitis-like skin lesion with IgE hyperproduction in NC/Nga mice. Int Immunol 1997;9:461–466.
9 Leung DYM: Atopic dermatitis: Immunobiology and treatment with immune modulators. Clin Exp Immunol 1997;107:25–30.
10 Watanabe N, Kobayashi A, Hirano T, Miyajima H, Ovary Z: Detection of IgE antibody-forming cells by passive cutaneous anaphylaxis using cell extract from lymphoid organs. J Immunol Methods 1987;96:41–45.
11 Grouls V, Helpap B: Selective staining of eosinophils and their immature precursors in tissue sections and autoradiographs with Congo red. Stain Technol 1981;56:323–325.
12 Matsuda H, Kitamura Y, Sonoda T, Imori T: Precursor of mast cell fixed in the skin of mice. J Cell Physiol 1981;108:409–415.
13 Matsuda H, Kawakita K, Kiso Y, Nakano T, Kitamura Y: Substance P induces granulocyte infiltration through degranulation of mast cells. J Immunol 1989;142:927–931.
14 Watanabe M, Tagami H, Horii H, Takahashi M, Klingman AM: Functional analyses of the superficial stratum corneum in atopic xerosis. Arch Dermatol 1991;127:1689–1692.
15 Imokawa G, Abe A, Jin K, Higaki Y, Kawashima M, Hidano A: Decreased level of ceramides in stratum corneum of atopic dermatitis: An etiologic factor in atopic dry skin? J Invest Dermatol 1991;96:523–526.
16 Ogawa M, Berger PA, McIntyre OR, Clendenning WE, Ishizaka K: IgE in atopic dermatitis. Arch Dermatol 1971;103:575–580.
17 Uehara M: Heterogeneity of serum IgE levels in atopic dermatitis. Acta Derm Venereol Suppl (Stockh) 1986;66:404–408.
18 Omoto M, Sugiura H, Uehara M: Histopathological features of recalcitrant erythema of the face in adult patients with atopic dermatitis. J Dermatol 1994;21:87–91.

International Archives of Allergy and Immunology

Int Arch Allergy Immunol 1999;120(suppl 1):76–81

Atopic Asthma Is Dominant in Elderly Onset Asthmatics: Possibility for an Alteration of Mast Cell Function by Aging through Fc Receptor Expression

Ryo Atsuta[a,b] Kazuo Akiyama[d] Takuji Shirasawa[c] Ko Okumura[b]
Yoshinosuke Fukuchi[a] Chisei Ra[b]

Departments of [a]Respiratory Medicine and [b]Immunology, Juntendo University School of Medicine, [c]Tokyo Metropolitan Institute of Gerontology, Tokyo, and [d]National Sagamihara Hospital, Sagamihara, Kanagawa, Japan

Key Words
Atopic asthma · Asthma, elderly onset · Fc receptor · Mast cell · IgE

Abstract
The morbidity and mortality of elderly onset asthma have recently been on the increase. To evaluate the allergic status of the elderly onset asthmatics, we performed skin tests for allergens and estimated serum total IgE levels of the patients. The proportion of the skin-test-positive patients among the elderly onset asthmatics was significantly larger than that in the younger onset group, whereas no significant difference was observed in the frequency of patients with serum total IgE levels higher than the normal range (287.2 IU/ml). On the other hand, in the experiments with aged mice, isolated peritoneal mast cells (PMC) showed a considerable decrease in the FcγRIIB/III expression and higher degranulation triggered by 2.4G2, as compared to the PMC derived from young mice. Since FcγRIIB has been shown to act as a negative regulator, we speculate that in the aged mice Fc receptor-mediated mast cell function may be upregulated by a release from the negative regulation as a result of decreased FcγRIIB expression. Our results obtained from a mouse model system may help to understand pathophysiological mechanisms underlying elderly onset asthma.

Introduction

Bronchial asthma is defined as a chronic inflammation accompanied by reversible airway obstruction and can be classified into two groups from the standpoint of the time of onset, namely onset in childhood and onset in adulthood. The morbidity and mortality of both groups have recently increased. For example, while 30 years ago the morbidity of bronchial asthma in infants and adults in Japan was 2–3 and 1–1.5%, respectively, recent research revealed that the morbidity increased to 3–7% in infants and to 3–4% in adults [1, 2]. Adult onset asthma can be further classified into two groups, younger onset and elderly onset asthma, and between these two types there are physiological and immunological differences. Asthma in the elderly is important, because the number of the asthmatics among the elderly has recently increased as a result of the general increase in age of our society. It has been reported that approximately 30% of the adult asth-

KARGER
Fax + 41 61 306 12 34
E-Mail karger@karger.ch
www.karger.com

1018–2438/99/1205–0076$17.50/0

Accessible online at:
http://BioMedNet.com/karger

Dr. Chisei Ra
Juntendo University School of Medicine
2-1-1 Hongo, Bunkyo-ku
Tokyo 113-8421 (Japan)
Tel. +81 3 5802 1591, Fax +81 3 3813 5512

matics are patients aged over 60 years in Japan [3], and that 12.4% are aged 65–74 years in America [4]. Furthermore, Akiyama [3] estimated that 2/3 of the cases of death due to asthma occurred in elderly patients, but pathophysiological mechanisms underlying asthma in the elderly are not yet well understood.

Even in the elderly, bronchial asthma is known to be caused by allergic reactions in which the high affinity IgE receptor (FcεRI) on the surface of effector cells, especially mast cells, plays a key role [5]. Binding of multivalent antigens to receptor-bound IgE on mast cells leads to an aggregation of multiple IgE receptor complexes, and subsequently induces degranulation and the release of inflammatory mediators such as histamine which are responsible for allergic symptoms. Mast cells also express Fc receptors for IgG, FcγRII and FcγRIII. In particular, the FcγRIIB has recently been shown to act as a negative regulator of immune-complex-triggered cell activation [6] and to regulate not only FcγRIII-mediated activation but also FcεRI-mediated reaction such as cellular degranulation and the release of mediators [7, 8]. Thus, it is possible that these three Fc receptors might be involved in molecular mechanisms of asthma through controlling mast cell function.

In order to understand the mechanisms of elderly onset asthma, we first performed the skin test for allergens and evaluated serum IgE levels. Positive cases for the skin test in elderly onset asthmatics were more frequent as compared to those in younger onset asthmatics, while no significant difference in the serum IgE levels was observed between the two groups.

Since these results suggest a mechanism by which aging alters the sensitivity of mast cells in the skin, we next examine the mast cell function in aged mice to test this possibility. We documented here that peritoneal mast cells (PMC) derived from aged mice were more sensitive to immunological stimulation and that this was negatively correlated with the amount of Fc receptor expression.

Materials and Methods

Participants

The 399 subjects included in this retrospective study were outpatients of the National Sagamihara Hospital and the Juntendo University Hospital, of whom 74 subjects were diagnosed as elderly onset asthmatics (over 60 years old) in 1991–1994 and 325 as younger onset asthmatics (under 60 years old). The diagnosis of asthma was made based on physical and laboratory examinations such as tests for bronchial hypersensitivity and reversibility, eosinophil counts in the provocation sputa and symptoms following the guideline of the Japanese Society of Allergology. We classified asthmatics by age at onset on the basis of their subjective symptoms and past histories. The allergic status was evaluated through the skin tests for allergens and the serum total/specific IgE levels. In this study, an elderly onset asthmatic was defined as a patient whose age at the onset was over 60.

Skin Tests for Allergens

Intradermal skin tests were carried out according to the intradermal injection technique employing Torii allergens (Torii, Tokyo, Japan). When the diameter of the erythema was over 20 mm or that of the wheal was over 10 mm, the reaction was judged positive for the allergen.

Evaluation of Serum Total/Specific IgE Levels

Serum total IgE levels were determined with a solid phase radioimmunoassay test (RIST) employing a RIST kit (Pharmacia, Uppsala, Sweden). Prevalence was estimated based on the presence of 400 IU/ml RIST or higher. The serum concentrations of the specific IgE to house dust, domestic mites, true fungi, and animal dander were determined for each sample by a radioallergosorbent test (RAST; Pharmacia). The results were presented at RAST scores. Prevalence was estimated on the basis of a RAST score of 2 or higher.

Animals

Female C57BL/6 mice were purchased from Japan SLC (Shizuoka, Japan). Mice were between 6 and 8 weeks old (young mice) or between 72 and 94 weeks (aged mice). The animals were housed in groups of 10 at 25 °C with a 12-hour light/dark cycle. Food and water were available ad libitum.

Purification of mouse PMC

Mouse PMC were obtained by lavaging the pleural and peritoneal cavities with 5 ml of TG buffer (Tyrode's buffer lacking calcium and magnesium, containing 0.1% gelatin). The peritoneal lavage was centrifuged at 500 *g* for 5 min at 4 °C. The cell pellet was resuspended in 1 ml of TG buffer (5 mice/ml), and layered on 2 ml of 22.5% metrizamide in TG buffer, and centrifuged at 450 *g* for 20 min at room temperature and the pellet was resuspended in PBS. Purity of PMC was over 90%.

Immunofluorescence Flow Cytometry

FcεRI on PMC (5×10^5) was saturated with mouse IgE (Pharmingen, San Diego, Calif., USA) in 100 µl of PBS on ice for 40 min, and after washing was subsequently treated with FITC-conjugated monoclonal antibody against mouse IgE (Pharmingen) for 40 min on ice. For FcγRIIB and FcγRIII, PMC were treated with FITC-conjugated rat anti-mouse FcγRIIB/III monoclonal antibody, 2.4G2 (Pharmingen). Flow-cytometric analysis was performed on a FACScan flow cytometer (Becton Dickinson, Oxnard, Calif., USA). Data were illustrated using a CELL Quest Software (Becton Dickinson Immunochemistry System, Oxnard, Calif., USA).

Degranulation of PMC

Degranulation of mast cells was estimated as described previously [9]. Briefly, 0.25 ml of cell suspension (1×10^5 cells) in fresh RPMI medium (Nissui Pharmaceutical Co., Tokyo, Japan) was incubated at 37 °C for 20 min without shaking. Samples were then incubated with biotinylated 2.4G2 (0.4 µg/ml) at 37 °C for 15 min, and subsequently incubated with avidin (4 µg/ml) for 5 min at 37 °C. The reaction was stopped by cooling the samples on ice for 10 min, and a drop (0.03 ml) of 0.1% toluidine blue was added to each sample, and degranulated mast cells were counted (over 500 mast cells per sample) under light microscopy. Results are expressed as the percentage of the degranulated mast cells.

Statistical Analysis

Statistical analyses have been carried out where indicated, using Fisher's contingency analysis.

Results and Discussion

Many epidemiological surveys have revealed that there are two peaks of the asthma prevalence when plotted against the actual age of the asthmatics: one is found in childhood and another in adulthood [10]. A similar distribution was observed in the subjects we examined in this study, even if plotted against the age at onset of asthma. As demonstrated in figure 1, the first peak was found in children under the age of 9, and the second peak occurred in adults aged 40–49.

In order to examine the allergic status in elderly onset bronchial asthma, we first performed skin tests for allergens in all subjects. As shown in figure 2, the elderly onset asthmatics showed a significantly higher frequency of positive skin tests (except *Candida albicans*) than the younger onset asthmatics ($p < 0.05$): there were 49 positive cases (66.2%) among the 74 elderly onset asthmatics compared with 174 cases (53.5%) among the 325 younger onset asthmatics. In contrast to our observation, Barbee et al. [11] reported that the proportion of positive skin tests for main allergens tended to decrease with aging. This discrepancy may be due to a difference in the classification method. Whereas in most of the previous studies asthmatics were classified by the actual age of the patients, we classified the patients according to the age of onset of asthma in the present study. Our results of the skin tests indicate that the atopic type is dominant in the elderly onset asthmatics compared with the younger onset asthmatics.

We next examined serum total IgE levels in all subjects. The distribution of serum total IgE levels revealed that the maximal peak was found in youth, and the second peak at around 50 years of age and then it tended to decrease with aging (data not shown). Similar results were reported by Hanneuse et al. [12]. The distribution of serum total IgE levels of elderly onset asthmatics was demonstrated in figure 3. The mean IgE level of 74 elderly onset asthmatics was 287.2 IU/ml, 15 cases (20.3%) were over 400 IU/ml and 5 cases (6.8%) over 1,000 IU/ml. With regard to antigen-specific IgE levels, there were 16 positive cases (21.6%) for the IgE against true fungi and 19 positive cases (25.7%) for the IgE against house dust.

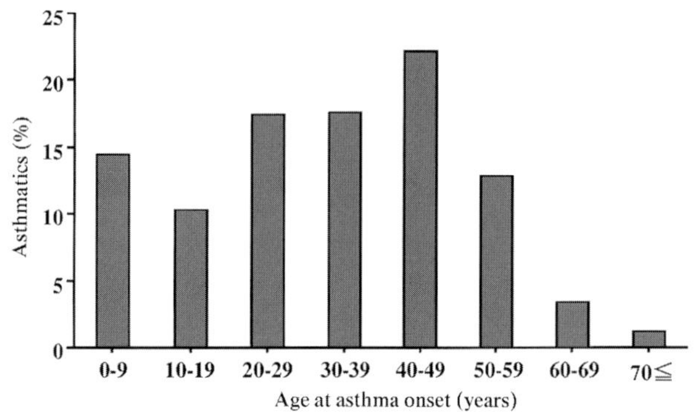

Fig. 1. Distribution of outpatients at the National Sagamihara Hospital according to age at onset of asthma.

Yokota et al. [13] reported similar results in which 30–50% of elderly onset asthmatics had more than 400 IU/ml of serum total IgE and the mean was 250–400 IU/ml in the asthmatics older than 60 years.

We next investigated the relationship between the frequency of positive skin tests and serum total IgE levels in elderly onset asthmatics. In contrast to the higher frequency of positive skin tests in elderly onset asthmatics, no significant difference was observed when we compared the IgE levels in the elderly onset asthmatics with those in the younger onset asthmatics (fig. 2); there were 15 positive cases (20.3%) among 74 elderly onset asthmatics compared with 63 positive cases (19.4%) among 325 younger onset asthmatics. The discrepancy of the positive rate between skin tests and serum total IgE levels suggests the possibility that an additional factor characterizes the immediate type hypersensitivity in the elderly onset bronchial asthma.

Bronchial asthma is known to be caused by an allergic response, which is initiated by Fc receptors, especially FcεRI on mast cells [14, 15]. As an initial approach to analyzing the molecular mechanisms of the elderly onset bronchial asthma, we examined the influence of aging on Fc receptor expression in mast cells. In this study, aged and young mice were compared as a model system. PMC were collected from 72- to 96-week-old (aged) and 6- to 8-week-old (young) mice and examined for the expression of the Fc receptors. Mouse mast cells express three kinds of Fc receptors, namely FcεRI, FcγRIIB and FcγRIII. Expression of these receptors on the cell surface was analyzed with a flow cytometer using IgE and anti-IgE antibody for FcεRI and 2.4G2 for FcγRIIB/III. As demonstrated in figure 4, PMC from the aged mice showed a

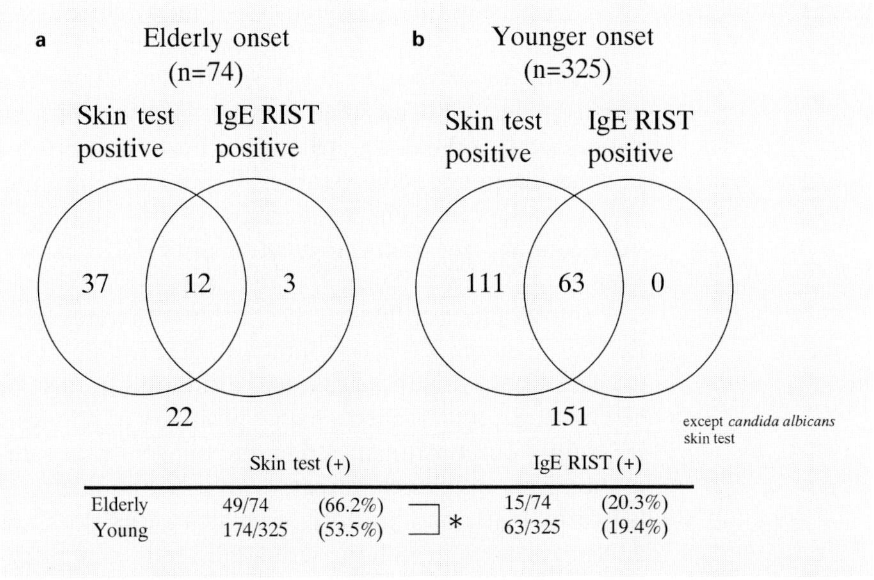

Fig. 2. Comparative analysis of immediate intradermal reaction and serum total IgE levels in the elderly onset and younger onset asthmatics. Venn diagrams illustrate the spectrum of allergic status: allergic status in 74 elderly onset asthmatics (**a**) and 325 younger onset asthmatics (**b**). Skin tests were performed using major allergens except *Candida albicans.* Statistical analyses were carried out using Fisher's contingency analysis.

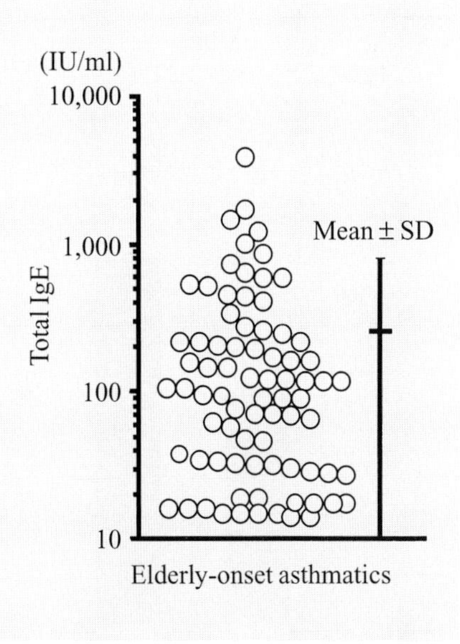

Fig. 3. Distribution of serum total IgE levels in the elderly onset asthmatics. The y-axis represents the log scale for IgE concentration. Seventy-four elderly onset asthmatics were examined for the concentration of serum IgE. The mean concentration was 287.2 IU/ml, and 15 cases were over 400 IU/ml and 5 cases over 1,000 IU/ml.

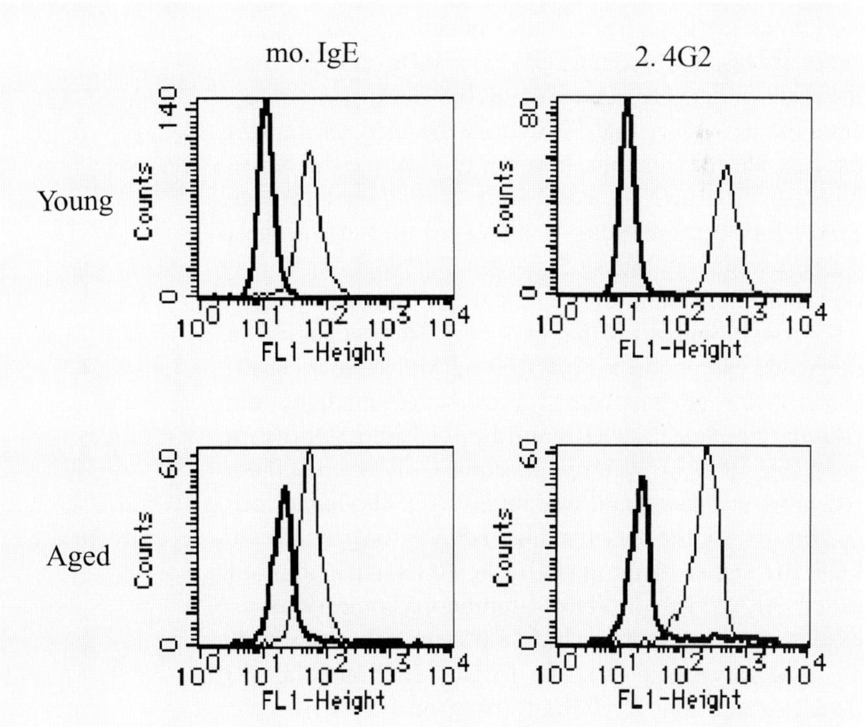

Fig. 4. Flow-cytometric analysis of Fc receptors expressed on PMC from aged mice and from young mice. PMC were collected from 6- to 8-week-old (young) and 72- to 96-week-old mice (aged). For analysis of FcεRI, cells were saturated with mouse IgE, and subsequently incubated with (thin line) or without FITC-labeled anti-mouse IgE (bold line); for FcγRII and FcγRIII, cells were incubated with (thin line) or without FITC-labeled 2.4G2 (bold line). Representative data from five independent experiments were displayed.

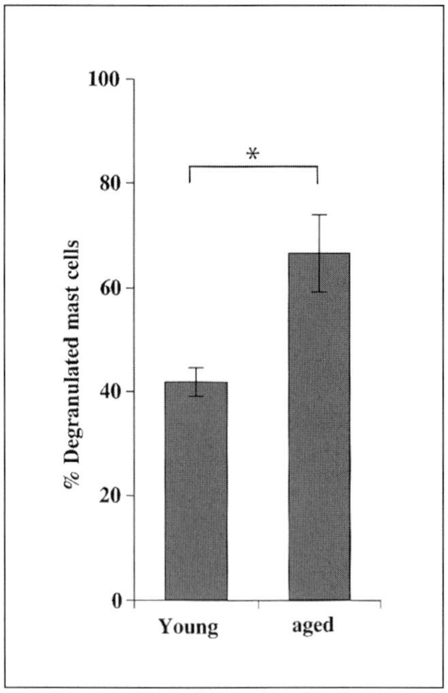

Fig. 5. FcγR-mediated degranulation of PMC from young mice and from aged mice. PMC from 6- to 8-week-old (young) and 72- to 96-week-old mice (aged) were incubated with biotinylated 2.4G2, and subsequently triggered with avidin. The results are shown as mean values ± SD from three independent experiments.

remarkably decreased level of FcγRIIB/III expression as compared to those from young mice, whereas a small decrease was observed in FcεRI expression on PMC from the aged group. Decreased FcγRIIB/III expression suggests the possibility that PMC from the aged mice might have an altered function. In order to examine this possibility, FcγRIIB/III on PMC were cross-linked through 2.4G2 for degranulation. As displayed in figure 5, mast cells derived from the aged group had greater degranulation than those from the young group through FcγR ($p < 0.05$, $n = 3$), suggesting that in the aged mouse possibly a decreased expression of FcγRIIB on PMC led to the higher activation of mast cells, especially IgG-mediated degranulation. Since FcγRIIB and FcγRIII were not distinguishable in our assay, it remains unknown which of these receptors decreased and was involved in the higher cell activation. At the moment, we believe that it may be FcγRIIB rather than FcγRIII. FcγRIIB have a motif called AENTITY or ITIM (immunoreceptor tyrosine-based inhibition motif) which intracellularly transduces an inhibitory signal [16, 17]. In fact, Daëron et al. [7] demonstrated that FcγRIIB transfected into RBL cells inhibited FcγR-dependent cell activation. Conversely, FcγRIIB-deficient mice demonstrated an enhanced passive cutaneous anaphylactic reaction mediated by IgG [18]. These reports suggest that FcγRIIB acts as a general negative regulator of immune-complex-triggered cell activation and that the downregulation of FcγRIIB functions in enhancing mast cell activation. We therefore propose that the enhancement of degranulation of PMC from aged mice could be due to downregulation of FcγRIIB expression.

In most of the previous studies, asthmatics were classified based on the actual age of the patients. In this study, we classified asthmatics according to the age at onset of asthma and demonstrated a higher positivity of skin tests im elderly onset asthmatics than in younger onset asthmatics. This difference in the positive rate of skin tests between elderly and younger onset asthmatics does not appear to correlate with the serum IgE levels, which suggests the involvement of a factor other than IgE in elderly onset asthma. In our mouse model system, PMC isolated from the aged mice actually had a decreased level of FcγR expression on the cell surface and increased sensitivity for mast cell activation. These results suggest a mechanism through which aging affects mast cell function by an altered expression of the Fc receptors. Although further studies are required to address the relevance of our results obtained in the mouse model for the human system, our observations may provide an insight into mechanisms underlying bronchial asthma in the elderly.

References

1 Akiyama K: Review of epidemiological studies on adult bronchial asthma in Japan. Nippon Kyobu Shikkan Gakkai Zasshi 1994;32:200–210.

2 Sano Y: Epidemiology of asthma. Nippon Naika Gakkai Zasshi 1996;85:168–173.

3 Akiyama K: Adult bronchial asthma in Japan. Nippon Kyobu Shikkan Gakkai Zasshi 1991; 29:984–992.

4 Evans R 3d, Mullally DI, Willson RW, Gergen PJ, Rosenberg HM, Grauman JS, Cheverley FM, Feinleib M: National trends in the morbidity and mortality of asthma in the US. Prevalence, hospitalization and death from asthma over two decades: 1965–1984. Chest 1987;91: 65–74.

5 Ravetch JV, Kinet J: Fc receptors. Annu Rev Immunol 1991;9:457–492.

6 Fridman WH: Regulation of B-cell activation and antigen presentation by Fc receptors. Curr Opin Immunol 1993;5:355–360.

7 Daëron M, Bonnerot C, Latour S, Fridman WH: Murine recombinant FcγRIII, but not FcγRII, trigger serotonin release in rat basophilic leukemia cells. J Immunol 1992;149: 1365–1373.

8 Daëron M, Malbec O, Latour S, Arock M, Fridman WH: Regulation of high-affinity IgE receptor-mediated mast cell activation by murine low-affinity IgG receptors. J Clin Invest 1995; 95:577–585.

9 Daëron M, Duc HT, Kanellopoulos J, Le Bouteiller P, Kinsky R, Voisin GA: Allogenic mast cell degranulation induced by histocompatibility antibodies: An in vitro model of transplantation anaphylaxis. Cell Immunol 1975;20:133–155.

10 Burney PGJ: Epidemiologic trends; in Barnes PJ, Grunstein MM, Leff AR, Woolcock AJ (eds): Asthma. New York, Lippincott-Raven, 1997, vol 1, pp 35–47.

11 Barbee R, Kaltenhorn W, Lebowitz MD, Burrows B: Longitudinal changes in allergen skin test reactivity in a community population sample. J Allergy Clin Immunol 1987;79:16–24.

12 Hanneuse Y, Delespesse G, Hudson D, de Halleux F, Jacques JM: Influence of ageing on IgE-mediated reactions in allergic patients. Clin Allergy 1978;8:165–174.

13 Yokota S, Mitsunobu F, Mifune T, Hosaki Y, Ashida K, Tsugeno H, Tanizaki Y: Age-related changes of IgE-mediated allergic reaction in patients with late onset asthma – Relationship between IgE-mediated allergy and age at onset. Nippon Ronen Igakkai Zasshi 1998;35:367–373.

14 Blank U, Ra C, Miller L, White K, Metzger H, Kinet JP: Complete structure and expression in transfected cells of high affinity IgE receptor. Nature 1989;337:187–189.

15 Ra C, Jouvin MH, Vercelli D: Complete structure of the mouse mast cell receptor for IgE (Fc epsilon RI) and surface expression of chimeric receptors (rat-mouse-human) on transfected cells. J Biol Chem 1989;264:15323–15327.

16 Daëron M, Latour S, Marbec O, Espinosa E, Pina P, Pasmans S, Fridman WH: The same tyrosine-based inhibition motif, in the intracytoplasmic domain of FcγRIIB, regulates negatively BCR-, TCR-, and FcR-dependent cell activation. Immunity 1995;3:635–646.

17 Fridman WH, Bonnerot C, Daëron M, Amigorena S, Teillaud JL, Stautes C: Structural bases of Fcγ receptor functions. Immunol Rev 1992;125:49–76.

18 Takai T, Ono M, Hikida M, Ohmori H, Ravetch JV: Augmented humoral and anaphylactic responses in FcγRII-deficient mice. Nature 1996;379:346–349.

International Archives of
Allergy and Immunology

Int Arch Allergy Immunol 1999;120(suppl 1):82–85

Correlation between Respiratory Function and Airway Inflammation in Asthma

Tadanori Hashimoto Kenji Minoguchi Yasurou Kohno Kiyoko Wada
Kana Ueno Hideko Kobayashi Masahide Miyamoto Mitsuru Adachi

First Department of Internal Medicine, Showa University, Tokyo, Japan

Key Words

Sputum · Eosinophils · Peak expiratory flow · Forced expiratory volume in 1 s · Airway hyperresponsiveness

Abstract

Background: Eosinophilic airway inflammation is thought to be associated with airflow limitation and airway hyperresponsiveness. ***Methods:*** Spirometry, peak expiratory flow (PEF) measurement, histamine challenge test, and sputum induction with hypertonic saline inhalation were performed in 70 asymptomatic patients with asthma who were treated with bronchodilators or an inhaled corticosteroid (beclomethasone dipropionate, 400–800 μg/day) or both for more than 2 months. The relationships between the sputum eosinophils, respiratory function, and airway responsiveness to histamine were investigated. ***Results:*** Induced sputum was obtained from 53 patients. Although significant correlations between sputum eosinophils and forced expiratory volume in 1 s/forced vital capacity × 100% (FEV_1%) or maximum expiratory flow at 25% of the forced vital capacity ($\dot{V}_{25}$) divided by height ($\dot{V}_{25}$/Ht) were observed, no significant correlations were found between sputum eosinophils and percent predicted PEF (%PEF) or airway responsiveness to histamine. Furthermore, airway responsiveness to histamine was not correlated with FEV_1%, $\dot{V}_{25}$/Ht or %PEF. ***Conclusion:*** Single-point measurements of FEV_1% and $\dot{V}_{25}$/Ht but not PEF or airway responsiveness to histamine correlate with the degree of airway inflammation evaluated indirectly with induced sputum.

Introduction

Guidelines for the management of chronic asthma recommend monitoring of asthma symptoms and respiratory function by spirometry or peak expiratory flow (PEF) [1]. On the basis of these findings, the severity of asthma is determined and the appropriate long-term anti-inflammatory treatment is given.

Noninvasive assessment of airway inflammation in asthma has been a focus of interest for the last 10 years. Although several techniques, such as measurement of serum eosinophil cationic protein, exhaled nitric oxide, bronchoalveolar lavage and bronchial biopsy, have been developed, analysis of induced sputum is particularly useful because it is noninvasive, repeatable, and can be performed in outpatient clinics [2]. Because eosinophils in

KARGER

Fax + 41 61 306 12 34
E-Mail karger@karger.ch
www.karger.com

1018–2438/99/1205–0082$17.50/0

Accessible online at:
http://BioMedNet.com/karger

Kenji Minoguchi, MD, PhD
First Department of Internal Medicine
Showa University, School of Medicine, 1-5-8
Hatanodai, Shinagawa-ku, Tokyo 142 (Japan)
Tel. +81 3 3784 8532, Fax +81 3 3784 8742

induced sputum may correlate with airway eosinophilia, airway inflammation can be monitored [3].

To determine which variables of respiratory function indirectly correlate with airway inflammation evaluated by induced sputum in asthma, in the present study we examined the relationship between sputum eosinophils and respiratory function, including forced expiratory volume in 1 s/forced vital capacity (FVC) × 100% (FEV_1%), percent predicted PEF (%PEF), maximum expiratory flow at 25% of the FVC divided by height ($\dot{V}_{25}$/Ht), and airway responsiveness to histamine at a single-point measurement.

Material and Methods

Subjects

Seventy patients with asthma (38 women and 32 men), aged 18–65 years, were studied. All patients were treated with bronchodilators (slow-release theophylline with or without an oral β_2-agonist) or an inhaled corticosteroid (beclomethasone dipropionate, 400–800 µg/day) or both. No patients had asthma symptoms or had a respiratory infection in the 8 weeks before examination. Informed consent was obtained before the study.

Study Design

This was a cross-sectional study. Clinical conditions, including asthma symptoms and twice daily PEF recording at home with a mini-Wright peak flow meter, were monitored for more than 2 months before enrollment. On arrival, PEF values, spirometric values, histamine challenge test, and sputum induction with hypertonic saline inhalation were performed at approximately the same time each day. All bronchodilators were withheld for at least 12 h and inhaled corticosteroids were withheld for at least 24 h before examinations. Plasma concentrations of theophylline in subjects receiving this drug were measured before examinations and were confirmed to be less than 5 µg/ml.

Respiratory Function

Respiratory function was measured 3 times with a spirometer, and the highest values of the three measurements were expressed. The PEF was expressed as the best value of three measurements, and %PEF was calculated according to the standard data of healthy Japanese subjects [4].

Airway Responsiveness to Histamine

Bronchial responsiveness to histamine was measured. Patients inhaled doubling concentrations of histamine administered with an ultrasonic nebulizer (DeVilbis, Somerset, Pa., USA) for 2 min by tidal breathing. Increasing concentrations of histamine were administered until FEV_1 decreased by at least 20% from baseline values. Results are expressed as the provocative concentration that caused a 20% decrease in FEV_1 from baseline (PC_{20}).

Sputum Induction and Processing

Sputum induction was performed as described previously [5]. Briefly, sputum was induced by inhalation of increasing concentrations of hypertonic saline (0.9, 1.8, 3, 4 and 5%) until an adequate sample was collected. Patients were encouraged to cough deeply after each inhalation. Cell plugs in sputum were separated from saliva and treated with Wright-Giemsa stain so that inflammatory cells could be counted. The percentage of inflammatory cells was determined by counting 900 cells under a light microscope.

Table 1. Patient characteristics (n = 53)

	Values
Male/female	24/29
Mean age, years	42.4±2.0
Atopy/nonatopy	27/26
Duration, months	70.3±13.7
Respiratory function	
PEF, l/min	437.0±11.6
% PEF	83.5±1.8
FVC, l	2.94±0.1
%FVC	90.8±2.6
FEV_1, l	2.25±0.08
FEV_1 %	76.2±1.2
$\dot{V}_{25}$, l/s	0.98±0.07
$\dot{V}_{25}$/Ht, l/s/m	0.60±0.04
PC_{20}, µg/ml	863.5±203.5
Induced sputum, %	
Eosinophils	22.9±2.3
Neutrophils	33.9±2.6
Lymphocytes	4.5±1.0
Macrophages	39.1±2.7

Statistical Analysis

log-transformed values of PC_{20} were used for analysis. Correlations were determined with the Fisher z test. Data are expressed as mean ± SEM, and differences with a p value <0.05 were considered significant.

Results

Induced sputum was obtained from 53 of the 70 patients with asthma (75.7%). Patient characteristics are summarized in table 1. Sputum eosinophils were negatively correlated with FEV_1% ($r = -0.446$, $p < 0.01$) and $\dot{V}_{25}$/Ht ($r = -0.460$, $p < 0.01$) (fig. 1). However, they were not correlated with either %PEF or histamine PC_{20} (fig. 1). Furthermore, histamine PC_{20} was not correlated with FEV_1% or $\dot{V}_{25}$/Ht (fig. 2). Sputum macrophages was correlated with only FEV_1% ($r = 0.466$, $p < 0.05$, data not shown). Sputum neutrophils or lymphocytes was not correlated with respiratory function or histamine PC_{20} (data not shown).

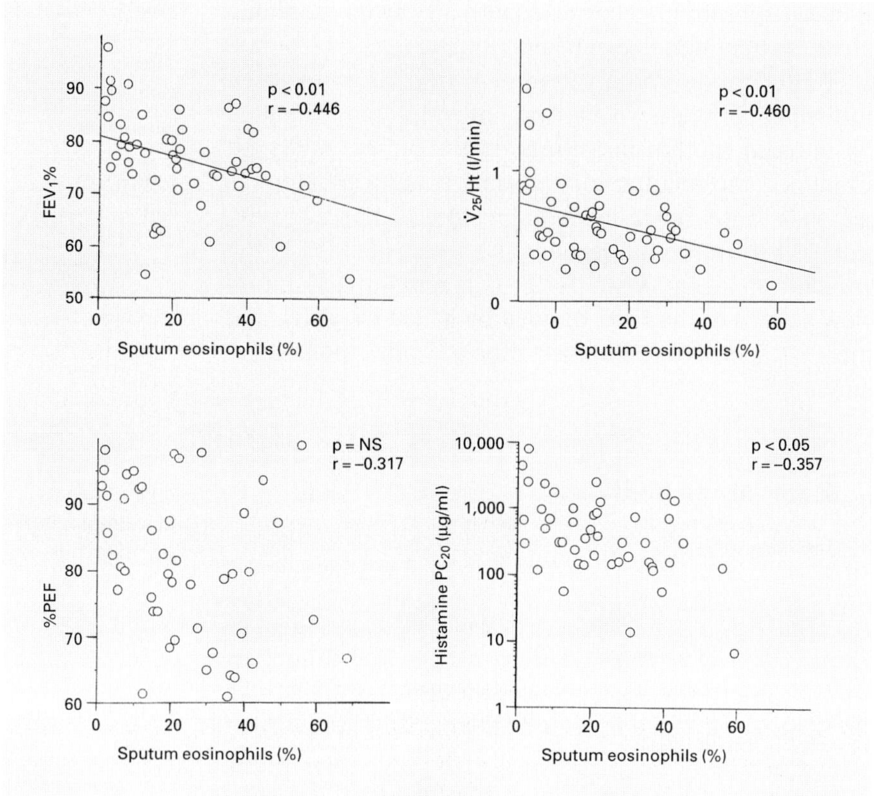

Fig. 1. Correlation between sputum eosinophils and FEV_1%, $\dot{V}_{25}$/Ht, %PEF or histamine PC_{20}. NS = Not significant.

Discussion

In the present study, we found a weak but significant correlation of sputum eosinophils with FEV_1% or $\dot{V}_{25}$/Ht but not with PEF values in asymptomatic patients with asthma. Furthermore, single measurements of airway responsiveness to histamine did not correlate with sputum eosinophils or respiratory function.

Bronchial asthma is defined as persistent airway inflammation that is associated with airflow limitation and respiratory symptoms. Although several studies have demonstrated that baseline respiratory function correlates weakly with the presence of the airway inflammatory cells, including eosinophils, mast cells, and activated T cells [6–8], other reports have failed to demonstrate a significant relationship [9]. In fact, we also observed a weak correlation of sputum eosinophils with baseline FEV_1 but not with PEF. One possible explanation for this weak correlation is that the collection of sputum with hypertonic saline induction does not accurately reflect airway inflammation. Another possible explanation is the presence of irreversible pathological changes, so-called airway remodeling, in the patients in this study.

There was a direct relationship between the number of sputum macrophages and baseline FEV_1 but not with PEF. A close relationship between FEV_1 and macrophages in sputum or BAL was also reported by Crimi et al. [10]. Because the role of macrophages in airway inflammation has not been fully investigated, further studies are necessary to elucidate it.

Current guidelines for the management of chronic asthma recommend that PEF be monitored as an objective marker of large airway dilatation. In the present study, we could not find a significant correlation between PEF and sputum eosinophils. Indeed, an increase in sputum eosinophils was still detected in some patients whose PEF readings were more than 80% of the predicted values. Although PEF reflects mainly a large airway dilatation, FEV_1 reflects from large to small airway dilatation. In fact, some patients with asthma show normal PEF values but data of FEV_1 are decreased. Therefore, FEV_1 may be more sensitive to reflecting the changes in the small airways than PEF. This possibility is also supported by the finding that $\dot{V}_{25}$/Ht, a marker of small airway dilatation, was negatively correlated with sputum eosinophils.

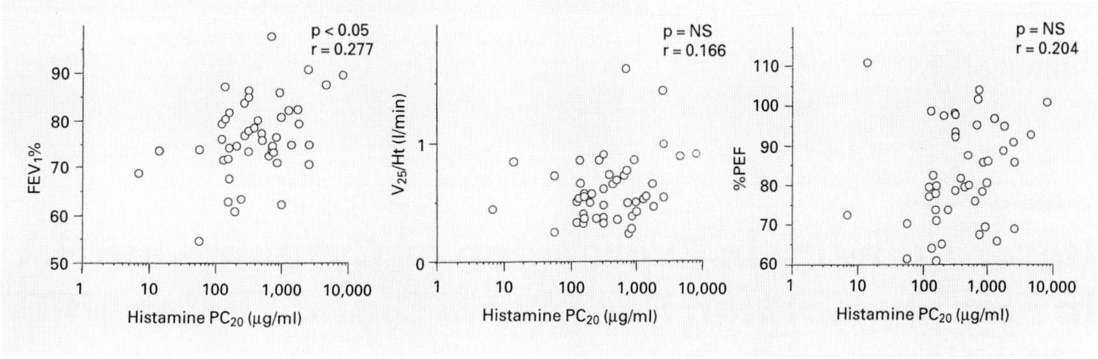

Fig. 2. Correlation between histamine PC_{20} and FEV_1%, $\dot{V}_{25}$/Ht or %PEF. NS = Not significant.

The relationship between airway responsiveness and the degree of airway inflammation is controversial. Some studies have demonstrated a close relationship [11–13], but others have not done so [10, 14, 15]. We did not find significant correlations between airway responsiveness and respiratory function or sputum eosinophils, perhaps because airway responsiveness is not regulated only by airway inflammation but may also be influenced by airway remodeling or other unknown factors, including autonomic dysfunction and genetic conditions.

Our present results suggest that single-point spirometric measurements weakly but significantly correlate with the degree of airway inflammation in asthma. Furthermore, single-point measurements of airway responsiveness do not indirectly correlate with the degree of airway inflammation. Therefore, respiratory function in asthma should be monitored by spirometry together with asthma symptoms and PEF monitoring.

References

1 National Asthma Education Program: Expert Panel Report 2: Guideline for the Diagnosis and Management of Asthma. Bethesda, National Institutes of Health, 1997, Publication No 98-4051.

2 Pizzichini E, Pizzichini MMM, Efthimiadis A, Evans S, Morriss MM, Squillace D, Gleich G, Dolovich J, Hargreave FE: Indices of airway inflammation in induced sputum: Reproducibility and validity of cell and fluid measurements. Am J Respir Crit Care Med 1996;154: 308–317.

3 Maestrelli P, Saetta M, Di Stefano A, Calcagni PG, Turato G, Ruggieri MP, Roggeri A, Mapp CE, Fabbri LM: Comparison of leukocyte counts in sputum, bronchial biopsies, and bronchoalveolar lavage. Am J Respir Crit Care Med 1995;152:1926–1931.

4 Tsukioka K: Peak expiratory flow in normal, healthy Japanese subjects. Kyowa Kikaku Tuushinn 1995;1:77–96.

5 Minoguchi K, Kohno Y, Oda N, Wada K, Miyamoto M, Yokoe T, Hashimoto T, Akabane T, Kobayashi H, Mita S, Kihara N, Adachi M: Effect of theophylline withdrawal on airway inflammation in asthma. Clin Exp Allergy 1998;28(suppl 3):57–63.

6 Bousquet J, Chanez P, Lacoste JY, Barneon G, Ghavanian N, Enander I, Venge P, Ahlstedt S, Simony-Lafontaine J, Godard P, Michel FB: Eosinophilic inflammation in asthma. N Engl J Med 1990;323:1033–1039.

7 Kirby JG, Hargreave FE, Gleich GJ, O'Byrne PM: Bronchoalveolar cell profiles of asthmatic and nonasthmatic subjects. Am Rev Respir Dis 1987;136:379–383.

8 Walker CM, Kaegi K, Braum P, Blaser K: Activated T cells and eosinophilia in bronchoalveolar lavages from subjects with asthma correlated with disease severity. J Allergy Clin Immunol 1991;88:935–942.

9 Jatakanon A, Lim S, Kharitonov SA, Chung KF, Barnes PJ: Correlation between exhaled nitric oxide, sputum eosinophils, and methacholine responsiveness in patients with mild asthma. Thorax 1998;53:91–95.

10 Crimi E, Spanevello A, Neri M, Ind PW, Rossi GA, Brusasco V: Dissociation between airway inflammation and airway hyperresponsiveness in allergic asthma. Am J Respir Crit Care Med 1998;157:4–9.

11 Wardlaw AJ, Dunnette S, Gleich GJ, Collins JV, Kay AB: Eosinophils and mast cells in bronchoalveolar lavage in subjects with mild asthma: Relationship to bronchial hyperreactivity. Am Rev Respir Dis 1988;137:62–69.

12 Walker C, Kaegi MK, Braum P, Blaser K: Activated T cells and eosinophilia in bronchoalveolar lavages from subjects with asthma correlated with disease severity. J Allergy Clin Immunol 1991;88:935–942.

13 Bradley BL, Azzawi M, Jacobson M, Assoufi B, Collins JV, Irani AM, Schwartz LB, Durham SR, Jeffery PK, Kay AB: Eosinophils, T-lymphocytes, mast cells, neutrophils, and macrophages in bronchial biopsy specimens from atopic subjects with asthma: Comparison with biopsy specimens from atopic subjects without asthma and normal control subjects and relationship to bronchial hyperresponsiveness. J Allergy Clin Immunol 1991;88:661–674.

14 Iredale MJ, Wankllin SAR, Phillips IP, Kraautstz T, Ind PW: Noninvasive assessment of bronchial inflammation in asthma: No correlation between eosinophilia of induced sputum and bronchial responsiveness to inhaled hypertonic saline. Clin Exp Allergy 1994;24: 940–945.

15 Rosi E, Ronchi MC, Grazzini M, Duranti R, Scano G: Sputum analysis, bronchial hyperresponsiveness, and airway function in asthma: Results of a factor analysis. J Allergy Clin Immunol 1999;103:232–237.

International Archives of Allergy and Immunology

Int Arch Allergy Immunol 1999;120(suppl 1):86–90

Heterogeneity in Expression of Cytokine mRNA in Freshly Isolated Peripheral Blood Eosinophils of Patients with Cutaneous-Disease-Associated Eosinophilia

Yutaka Hatano Kazumoto Katagiri Susumu Takayasu

Department of Dermatology, Oita Medical University, Oita, Japan

Key Words
Cytokines · Eosinophils · Eosinophilia

Abstract
Background: It is thought that there are subpopulations of eosinophils concerning cytokine production: some of them predominantly produce Th1 cytokines, while others produce Th2. ***Methods:*** By semiquantitative RT-PCR, the in vivo levels of the cytokine mRNA were measured in freshly isolated eosinophils and peripheral blood mononuclear cells (PBMCs) of 19 patients with eosinophilia, including 6 with atopic dermatitis, 4 with drug eruption, 1 with chronic dermatitis, 2 with erythroderma, 3 with bullous pemphigoid, 1 each with urticaria, adult T cell lymphoma, and hypereosinophilic syndrome, and 7 healthy individuals. Eosinophils and PBMCs were isolated by centrifugation over Ficoll-Paque and magnetic cell separation using anti-CD16 antibody. ***Results:*** The IL-4/IFN-γ ratio in eosinophils as well as PBMCs was increased and correlated well with IgE levels in atopic dermatitis. In other cytokines, such as IL-8, TNF-α and TGF-β_1, the levels of mRNA expression were variable among each sample. ***Conclusion:*** Not only helper T lymphocytes but also eosinophils may take part in the pathogenesis of cutaneous diseases by virtue of heterogeneity of Th1 and Th2 cytokine production.

Introduction

Eosinophils produce various cytokines [1–3]. Besides, cytokines synthesized by and stored in eosinophils, particularly Th2-type cytokines, may have autocrine effects such as increased cell survival in the tissue. Some previous studies have proposed the presence of distinct subpopulations of human eosinophils which express Th2 or Th1 cytokines [4, 5]. However, it remains unknown whether such heterogeneity is associated with the pathogenesis of diseases with eosinophilia. Thus, it would be interesting to know whether such heterogeneity is present in eosinophils in skin diseases. In the present study, we measured the levels of mRNA expression of various cytokines in peripheral blood eosinophils freshly isolated from patients with various cutaneous diseases with eosinophilia by means of semiquantitative RT-PCR. In addition, we compared the levels of mRNA expression by eosinophils with peripheral blood mononuclear cells (PBMCs) isolated simultaneously.

Materials and Methods

Study Population
A total of 19 patients having skin diseases with eosinophilia, i.e. 6 with atopic dermatitis (AD), 4 with drug eruption, 1 with chronic dermatitis, 2 with erythroderma, 3 with bullous pemphigoid (BP), 1 each with urticaria, adult T cell lymphoma and hypereosinophilic

KARGER
Fax + 41 61 306 12 34
E-Mail karger@karger.ch
www.karger.com

1018–2438/99/1205–0086$17.50/0

Accessible online at:
http://BioMedNet.com/karger

Yutaka Hatano
Department of Dermatology, Oita Medical University
1-1, Idaigaoka, Hasama-machi, Oita-gun
Oita 879-5593 (Japan)
Tel. +81 97 586 5822, Fax +81 97 586 5889

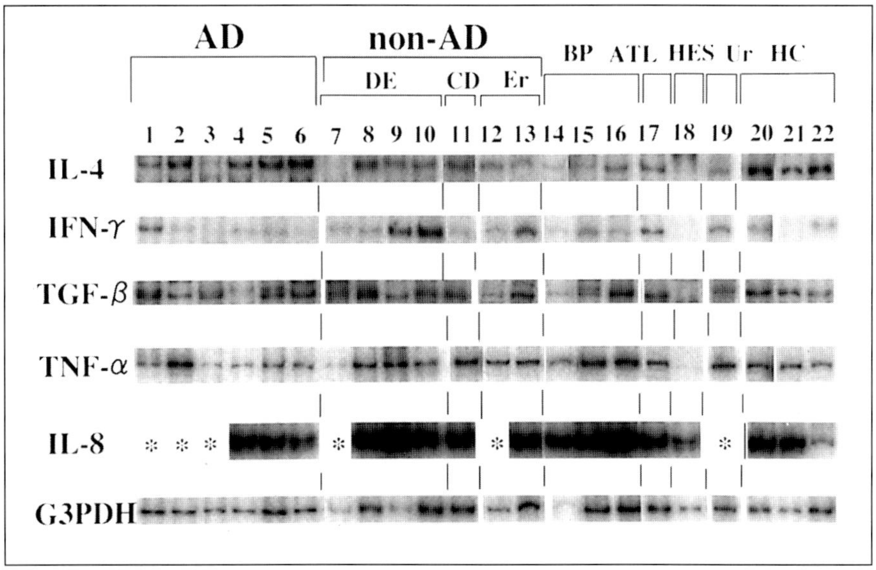

Fig. 1. Autoradiogram of PCR-assisted mRNA amplification for IL-4, IFN-γ, TGF-β, TNF-α, IL-8 and G3PDH in eosinophils from all subjects. DE = Drug eruption; CD = chronic dermatitis; Er = erythroderma; ATL = adult T cell lymphoma; Ur = urticaria; HC = healthy controls; * = measurement not performed.

syndrome (HES), and 7 healthy individuals were enrolled in this study after informed consent had been obtained. As a rule, eosinophils and PBMCs were isolated from the same blood sample. In 3 out of 7 healthy individuals, only eosinophils were isolated, and from 1 patient with erythroderma only PBMCs were obtained. Eosinophil counts ranged from 376 to 5,263/mm^3 (mean 1,387.8/mm^3), and serum levels of IgE ranged from 16 to 28,669 U/ml (mean 7,412 U/ml) in the patients. In all healthy individuals, both of these values were within normal ranges (less than 318/mm^3 and 350 U/ml, respectively). For analysis, we set 2 distinct disease groups. The Th1 disease group consisted of 7 patients with 'nonatopic dermatitis', including drug eruption, chronic dermatitis, and erythroderma (eosinophil count between 566 and 2,996/mm^3; levels of IgE between 58 and 11,805 U/ml, mean 2,639.8 U/ml). The group of Th2 diseases consisted of 6 patients with AD (eosinophil count from 376 to 1,185/mm^3, mean 604.7/mm^3; levels of IgE from 2,160 to 28,669 U/ml, mean 15,952.2 U/ml).

Preparation of Eosinophils and PBMCs

Eosinophils and PBMCs were isolated from the same blood sample. First, leukocytes were separated by sedimenting erythrocytes in heparinized blood with 6% Dextran 200000 (Wako). Then, mononuclear cells were isolated by centrifugation over Ficoll-Paque (Pharmacia). Next, eosinophils were separated by removing neutrophils by anti-CD16 monoclonal antibody (IgG1, 3G8, Funakoshi) and Dynabeads M-450 goat anti-mouse IgG (Dynal AS) after 0.87% ammonium chloride lysis of the remaining erythrocytes. The purity of the eosinophils was more than 97%. Isolated eosinophils and PBMCs were immediately homogenized in Isogen (Nippon Gene) that contained phenol and acid guanidinium thiocyanate. Total RNA was isolated by the acid guanidinium thiocyanate-phenol-chloroform method.

Semiquantitative RT-PCR

Spontaneous expression of mRNAs of several cytokines and glyceraldehyde-3-phosphate dehydrogenase (G3PDH) in freshly isolated eosinophils and PBMCs was measured by semiquantitative RT-PCR as described previously [6]. In brief, 50 ng of RNA was reverse-transcribed using random hexamers and MMLV reverse transcriptase (Gibco-BRL, Gaithersburg, Md., USA). The resultant cDNA was amplified by PCR with 1 μCi ^{32}P-dCTP. We performed PCR at the appropriate cycles (1 min at 94 °C, 1 min at 58 °C for IL-4 or at 60 °C for others, 1 min at 72 °C) within the linear amplification ranges as follows: 20 cycles for G3PDH, 24 cycles for IL-8, 28 cycles for IL-10, IFN-γ and TNF-α, 32 cycles for IL-4, and 34 cycles for IL-5 and TGF-β_1. The oligonucleotide primers for PCR were based on published mRNA sequences. Aliquots (1 μl) of each sample amplified with ^{32}P-dCTP were analyzed by electrophoresis on 5% acrylamide/Tris-borate EDTA gels and were subjected to autoradiography. DNA was quantified by phosphor image analysis (BAS2000; Fuji Medical Systems, Stanford, Conn., USA). For IL-5 and IL-10, PCR was performed only in eosinophils but not in PBMCs.

Statistical Analysis

The intensity of the amplified signals was normalized against G3PDH mRNA used as an internal standard. Results were evaluated using the Mann-Whitney U test only when study groups were composed of more than 5 samples. Correlation coefficients and statistical significance were determined using Spearman's correlation coefficient by rank. A level of $p < 0.05$ was considered statistically significant.

Results

Expression of Cytokine mRNA in Eosinophils

To eliminate the possibility that the amplified signals for each cytokine in eosinophils were due to contaminated PBMCs, RT-PCR was performed using a two-fold amount of RNA of contaminated PBMCs. Amplified signals for

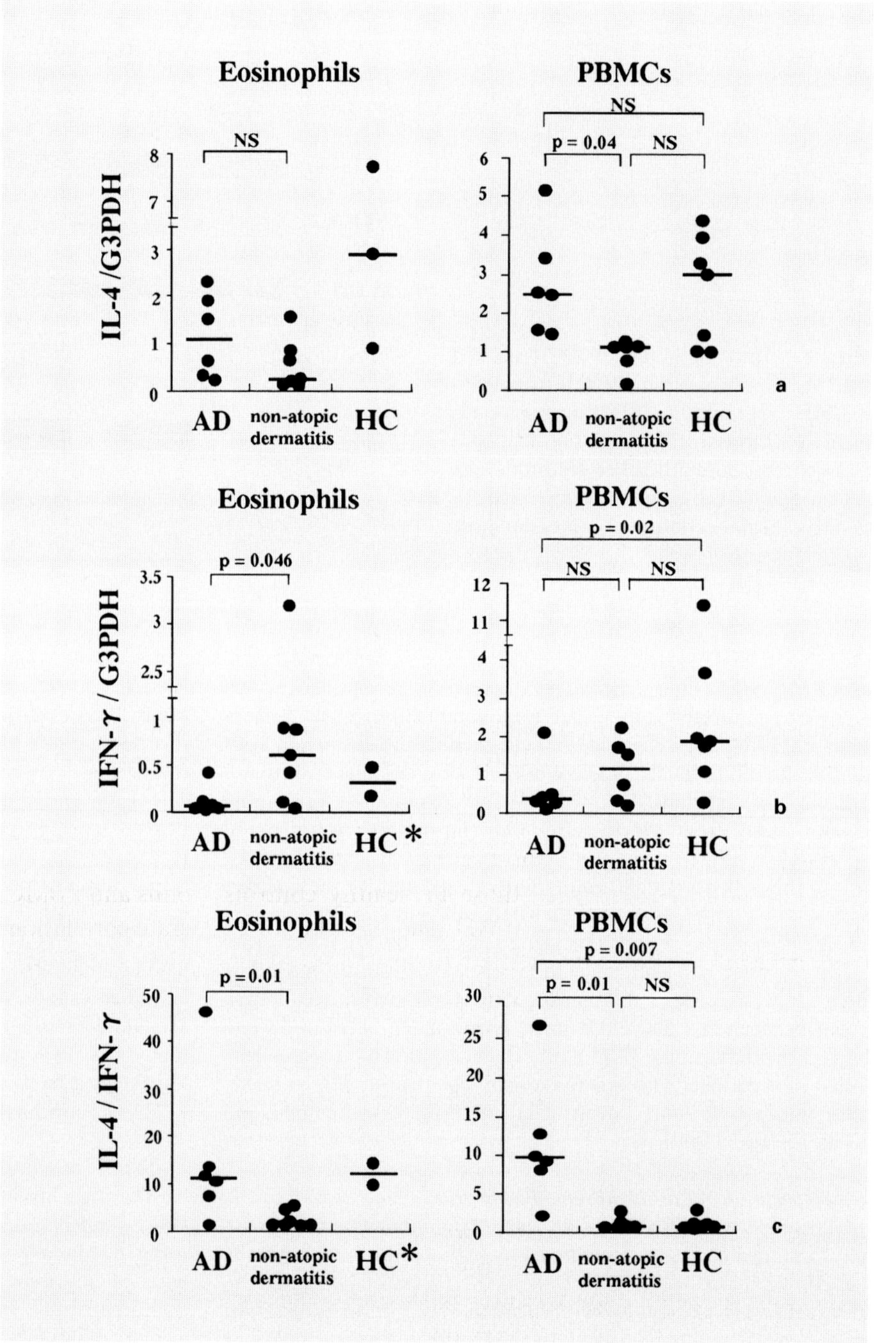

Fig. 2. Comparison of the expression of cytokine mRNA for (**a**) IL-4 and (**b**) IFN-γ, and of (**c**) IL-4/IFN-γ ratios in eosinophils and PBMCs from patients with AD, non-atopic dermatitis, and healthy controls (HC). The signal intensity of each cytokine was measured by phosphor image analysis and normalized against that of G3PDH. Medians are indicated by bold lines. Results were compared and evaluated using the Mann-Whitney U test. As in eosinophils, the group of healthy controls contained less than 5 samples, it was omitted in the statistical analysis. **b**, **c** In eosinophils, IFN-γ mRNA were detected in only 2 of 3 HC described. The ordinate indicates relative strength of photostimulated luminescence.

any cytokine were not detected (data not shown). Expressions of IL-4, IFN-γ, IL-8, TNF-α, and TGF-β_1 mRNA in eosinophils were detected in all of 19 patients and 3 healthy individuals, except for IFN-γ mRNA in 1 patient with HES and in 1 healthy individual (fig. 1). However, neither IL-5 nor IL-10 mRNA expression was detected in any individual. The levels of IL-8, TNF-α, and TGF-β_1 mRNAs were not statistically different between AD and nonatopic groups. The levels of IL-4 mRNA were also not statistically different between AD and nonatopic dermatitis, although they tended to be higher in the former (fig. 2a). In contrast, the levels of IFN-γ mRNA in AD were significantly decreased as compared with nonatopic dermatitis (fig. 2b).

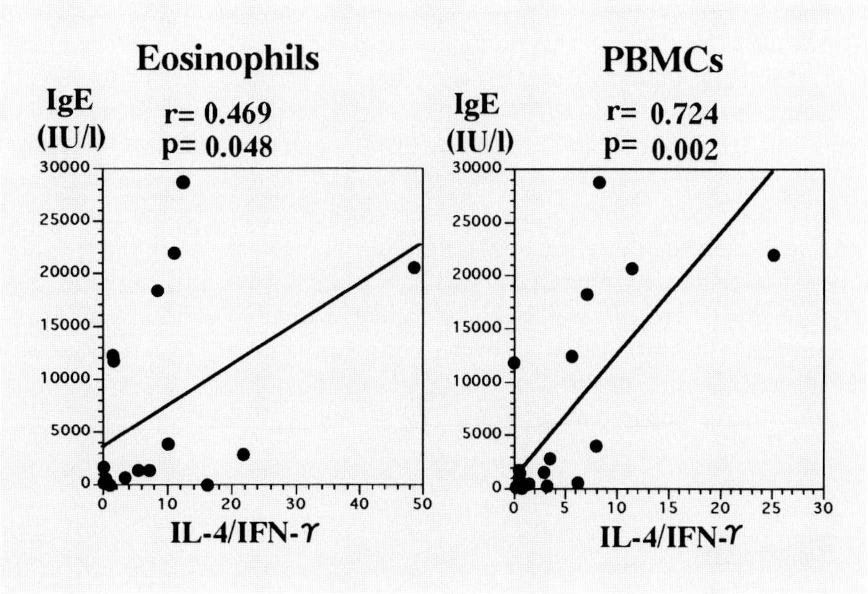

Fig. 3. Correlation between levels of IgE and the IL-4/IFN-γ ratio in eosinophils and PBMCs. A regression line is described in each graph. Results were evaluated using Spearman's correlation coefficient (r) by rank.

Expression of Cytokine mRNA in PBMCs

Expressions of mRNA of IL-4, IL-8, IFN-γ, TNF-α, and TGF-β_1 were detected in all samples (data not shown). The levels of IL-4 in AD were significantly increased as compared with those in nonatopic dermatitis, while not different from those in healthy controls (fig. 2a). The levels of IFN-γ in AD tended to be lower than those in nonatopic dermatitis, without statistical significance (fig. 2b), and were significantly decreased as compared with those in healthy controls (fig. 2b).

Correlation between IL-4/IFN-γ Ratio and IgE in Eosinophils and PBMCs

We examined the correlation between the IL-4/IFN-γ ratio and an IgE level which is a barometer of Th2 dominance, in order to know whether there exists a Th1/Th2 imbalance. Not only in PBMCs, but also in eosinophils, the IL-4/IFN-γ ratio significantly correlated with IgE (fig. 3). A stronger correlation was observed in PBMCs compared to eosinophils (fig. 3). Neither the other cytokines nor the ratio of their combinations correlated with the levels of IgE (data not shown). In both PBMCs and eosinophils, the IL-4/IFN-γ ratio in AD was significantly increased as compared with that in nonatopic dermatitis (fig. 2c). In PBMCs, the IL-4/IFN-γ ratio in AD was significantly increased as compared with that in healthy controls as well (fig. 2c).

Correlation of the mRNA Levels of Various Cytokines and the IL-4/IFN-γ Ratio between Eosinophils and PBMCs

There was no significant correlation in IL-4, IFN-γ, IL-8, TNF-α, and TGF-β_1 mRNA levels between eosinophils and PBMCs in any group (data not shown). A moderate correlation in the IL-4/IFN-γ ratio between eosinophils and PBMCs was detected (coefficient of correlation 0.41), although it was not statistically significant.

Discussion

It was reported that eosinophils isolated from healthy individuals are rarely able to express mRNA of cytokines except for IL-4 without stimulation [3]. However, in the present study, we could detect mRNA expression of IL-4, IFN-γ, IL-8, TNF-α, and TGF-β_1 without any stimulation in almost all samples. In contrast, IL-10 mRNA was not detected in eosinophils in our study, while it was detected in 2 of 7 samples in the previous study without stimulation [3]. These discrepancies may be attributed to the condition of PCR or to different sources of eosinophils, namely eosinophils from healthy individuals or from patients with cutaneous diseases and eosinophilia.

IL-4/IFN-γ ratios in both eosinophils and PBMCs correlated well with IgE levels in the present study, and they were increased in AD as compared with nonatopic dermatitis. These results suggest that eosinophils take part in the pathogenesis of cutaneous diseases with eosinophilia by expressing either Th1- or Th2- dominant cytokines. However, it remains unknown whether there is a cause-effect relationship between IL-4/IFN-γ imbalance in eosinophils and IgE production, although in PBMCs, such an imbalance has been known to induce IgE production [7]. In fact, a stronger correlation was observed in PBMCs with IgE levels than in eosinophils. Besides, the present study showed that peripheral eosinophilia was not always associated with Th2 diseases, since the patients with nonatopic dermatitis often showed severer eosinophilia than those with AD, although Th1 predominates in nonatopic dermatitis, as compared with AD.

No significant correlation in mRNA levels of the cytokines was found between eosinophils and PBMCs. This result suggests that mRNA expression of these cytokines in eosinophils may be regulated differently from those in PBMCs. At least the heterogeneous expression of the cytokine mRNA in peripheral eosinophils in our study may show that peripheral eosinophils associated with these skin diseases are already regulated before infiltrating into the inflamed tissues where they secrete cytokines and are destroyed. Further studies on the mechanism of regulation of cytokine production in eosinophils are required.

References

1 Silberstein DS: Eosinophil function in health and disease. Crit Rev Oncol Hematol 1995;19: 47–77.

2 Weller PF: Human eosinophils. J Allergy Clin Immunol 1997;100:283–287.

3 Nakajima H, Gleich GJ, Kita H: Constitutive production of IL-4 and IL-10 and stimulated production of IL-8 by normal peripheral blood eosinophils. J Immunol 1996;156:4859–4866.

4 Lamkhioued B, Aldebert D, Gounni AS, Delaporte E, Goldman M, Capron A, Capron M: Synthesis of cytokines by eosinophils and their regulation. Int Arch Allergy Immunol 1995; 107:122–123.

5 Lamkhioued B, Gounni AS, Aldebert D, Delaporte E, Prin L, Capron A, Capron M: Synthesis of type 1(IFN-γ) and type 2 (IL-4, IL-5, and IL-10) cytokines by human eosinophils. Ann NY Acad Sci 1996;796:203–208.

6 Katagiri K, Itami S, Hatano Y, Takayasu S: Increased levels of IL-13 mRNA, but not IL-4 mRNA, are found in vivo in peripheral blood mononuclear cells (PBMC) of patients with atopic dermatitis (AD). Clin Exp Immunol 1997;108:289–294.

7 Vercelli D, Jabara HH, Lauener RP, Geha RS: IL-4 inhibits the synthesis of IFN-gamma and induces the synthesis of IgE in human mixed lymphocyte cultures. J Immunol 1990;144: 570–573.

International Archives of Allergy and Immunology

Int Arch Allergy Immunol 1999;120(suppl 1):91–94

Difference in Apoptotic Function between Eosinophils from Peripheral Blood and Bronchoalveolar Lavage in Chronic Eosinophilic Pneumonia

Naoki Saita[a] Tohru Yamanaka[a] Hirotsugu Kohrogi[a] Masayuki Ando[a] Mitsuomi Hirashima[b]

[a]First Department of Internal Medicine, Kumamoto University, School of Medicine, Kumamoto, and
[b]Department of Immunology and Immunopathology, Kagawa Medical School, Kagawa, Japan

Key Words
Eosinophil chemotactic factor · Apoptosis · Eosinophilic pneumonia

Abstract
We compared apoptosis in eosinophils from bronchoalveolar lavage (BAL-Eos) with that in eosinophils from peripheral blood (PB-Eos) of 4 patients with chronic eosinophilic pneumonia (CEP). The survival rate of the BAL-Eos on the 3rd day of the culture was significantly higher than that of the PB-Eos (39.1 vs. 1.3%). The percentage of apoptotic cells in the PB-Eos after a 24-hour incubation was higher than that in the BAL-Eos (21.7 vs. 10.6%) according to an analysis with annexin V. We further found that ECF-PI9, an eosinophil chemotactic factor (ECF) derived from an established T cell line (STO-2), significantly suppressed the apoptosis of both PB-Eos and BAL-Eos and prolonged their survival. The expression of Fas on PB-Eos was significantly suppressed by ECF-PI9 (18.5 to 7.37%, $p < 0.05$), whereas ECF-PI9 failed to suppress the Fas expression on BAL-Eos (3.3 to 3.6%). In addition, an ECF with similar physicochemical properties and biological functions was isolated from the BAL fluid of patients with CEP. These data demonstrate differences between PB-Eos and BAL-Eos, and indicate that ECF-PI9 is involved in the pathogenesis of CEP.

Introduction

We have previously shown that patients with chronic eosinophilic pneumonia (CEP) can be divided into two groups according to the chemotactic response of their eosinophils from peripheral blood (PB-Eos) to an eosinophil chemotactic factor (ECF), ECF-PI9, derived from an established T cell line (STO-2) [1]. The classification using the chemotactic response may be a useful marker for the evaluation of therapy [2]. These results might reflect a functional heterogeneity of eosinophils in CEP.

CEP is characterized by the presence of an interstitial inflammatory reaction in the lung, and a large number of eosinophils in the PB and also in bronchoalveolar lavage (BAL) [3]. An increased production of interleukin 5 seems to be one of the critical pathophysiological features of CEP [4, 5], but the precise mechanism of eosinophil recruitment into the pulmonary space is not yet fully

KARGER

Fax + 41 61 306 12 34
E-Mail karger@karger.ch
www.karger.com

1018–2438/99/1205–0091$17.50/0

Accessible online at:
http://BioMedNet.com/karger

Dr. Naoki Saita
First Department of Internal Medicine
Kumamoto University, School of Medicine
1-1-1 Honjo
Kumamoto 860-0855 (Japan)

understood. Other chemical mediators might play a role in the pathogenesis of CEP. Eosinophils from BAL (BAL-Eos) differ from PB-Eos in their chemotactic response and eosinophil surface antigens [2, 6, 7]. Most of the eosinophils in alveolar spaces are in an activated state, as Nishikawa et al. [6] demonstrated, and in vitro studies have demonstrated that cell apoptosis decreases when the activation of inflammatory cells increases [8, 9]. Although several studies have been done on the correlation of eosinophils and apoptosis [10–12], there has been no comparison of eosinophil apoptosis in PB and BAL. The purpose of the present study was to clarify: (1) the kinetics of the apoptosis of PB- and BAL-Eos from CEP patients, and (2) the effect of ECF-PI9 on the apoptosis in these cells.

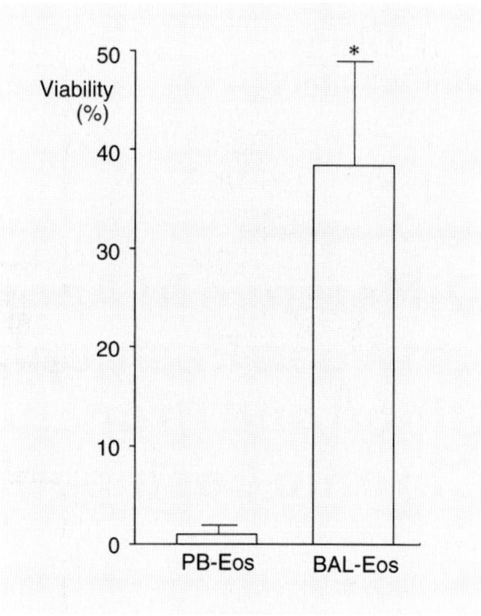

Fig. 1. Viability of PB-Eos and BAL-Eos after 3 days' culture. PB-Eos and BAL-Eos were cultured for 3 days and harvested. The viability of the eosinophils was evaluated by the trypan blue dye exclusion test. Data represent means ± SD of four cases (* $p < 0.01$).

Materials and Methods

Patients

The diagnosis of CEP was based on the patients' past history, physical examination, radiographic features, and the presence of increased numbers of eosinophils in lung tissue and BAL. Four CEP patients (age and sex: 56-year-old female, 43-year-old female, 45-year-old female and 57-year-old male) were examined.

Cell Fractionation

Peripheral blood leukocytes were obtained from heparinized venous blood. The separation of eosinophils was performed using a discontinuous density Percoll column (Pharmacia, Uppsala, Sweden) with five different concentrations, as previously described [1]. To remove residual neutrophils, we used a monoclonal antibody against CD16 in a negative and indirect selection procedure using immunomagnetic beads (Dynal, Oslo, Norway). BAL was performed in the involved lung segment. BAL fluid was centrifuged at 1,200 rpm for 10 min. Eosinophils from BAL were also enriched with a discontinuous density Percoll column, and the cells were suspended in 10% FCS-containing RPMI 1640 solution. In all cases, the eosinophil-rich fraction was more than 98% in purity, and the viability was greater than 99%.

Detection of Eosinophil Survival and Apoptosis

The viability of the eosinophils was evaluated by the trypan blue dye exclusion test after a 3-day incubation at 37°C in a 5% CO_2-containing incubator. The effects of ECF-PI9 on eosinophil survival were also assessed. The apoptosis of eosinophils was assessed with an annexin V FITC kit (Immunotech, Marseille, France) according to the methods of Levi-Schaffer et al. [13]. Briefly, eosinophils were cultured for 24 h in the presence or absence of ECF-PI9, harvested and washed with PBS by centrifugation for 3 min at 4,000 rpm. The cells were resuspended with 490 µl of binding buffer (10 m*M* Hepes, 140 m*M* NaCl, 2.5 m*M* $CaCl_2$, pH 7.4), and 1.25 µg propidium iodide and 5 ml of annexin V FITC solution were added. After 10 min incubation on ice, the cell sample was analyzed on a FACScan (Becton Dickinson, Mountain View, Calif., USA).

We also assessed the effects of ECF-PI9 on the Fas expression on eosinophils. PB-Eos and BAL-Eos were cultured for 24 h, and then the harvested cells were incubated with monoclonal antibodies against Fas (UB2, MBL, Nagoya, Japan) for 30 min. After washing, the cells were analyzed on the FACScan.

Results

In order to elucidate the survival rates of PB-Eos and BAL-Eos, the cells were cultured for 3 days, and viability was assessed by trypan blue dye exclusion. As shown in figure 1, the survival rate of BAL-Eos after 3 days' culture was significantly higher than that of PB-Eos (39.1 vs. 1.3%, $p < 0.01$). We further assessed the apoptosis of PB-Eos and BAL-Eos using the annexin V FITC kit after 24 h incubation. The percentages of apoptotic cells in PB-Eos and BAL-Eos were 21.7 and 10.6%, respectively (fig. 2a, b), suggesting that BAL-Eos were more resistant to apoptosis than PB-Eos. The effects of ECF-PI9 on eosinophil apoptosis were further elucidated. PB-Eos and BAL-Eos were cultured in the presence or absence of ECF-PI9 for 24 h. Thus, we found that ECF-PI9 suppressed eosinophil apoptosis and significantly prolonged eosinophil survival. When PB-Eos and BAL-Eos were cultured with ECF-PI9, the percentage of apoptotic cells in PB-Eos decreased from 21.7 to 9.2% with ECF-PI9 stimulation, and that of

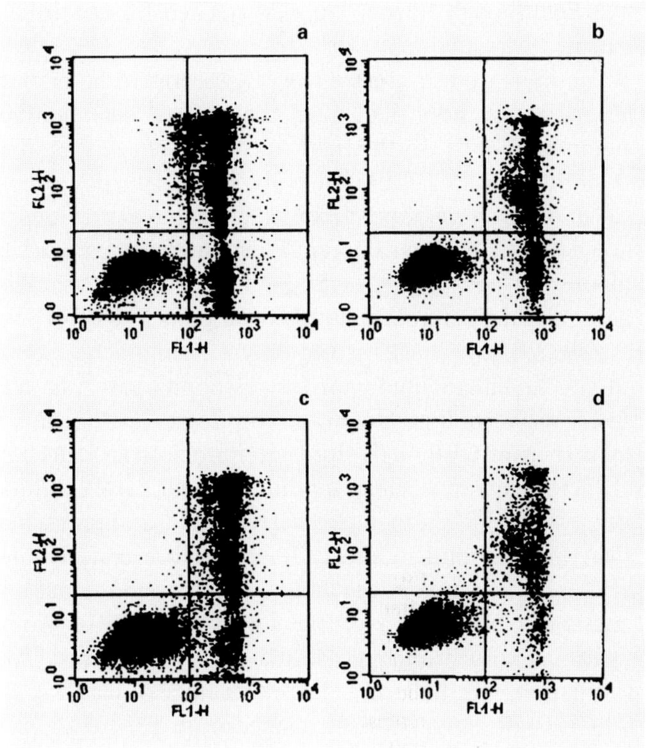

Fig. 2. Effects of ECF-PI9 on the apoptosis of PB-Eos and BAL-Eos. Eosinophils from PB (**a**, **b**) and BAL (**c**, **d**) of CEP patients were cultured for 24 h. The cells were harvested, and the rate of apoptosis was assessed with an annexin V FITC kit and analyzed on a FACScan. We also assessed the effect of ECF-PI9 on PB-Eos and BAL-Eos by culturing the cells with (**c**, **d**) or without (**a**, **b**) ECF-PI9. In each scan, the right upper quadrant shows necrosis, the left lower quadrant shows viable cells, and the right lower quadrant shows early apoptosis. One representative scan of four is shown.

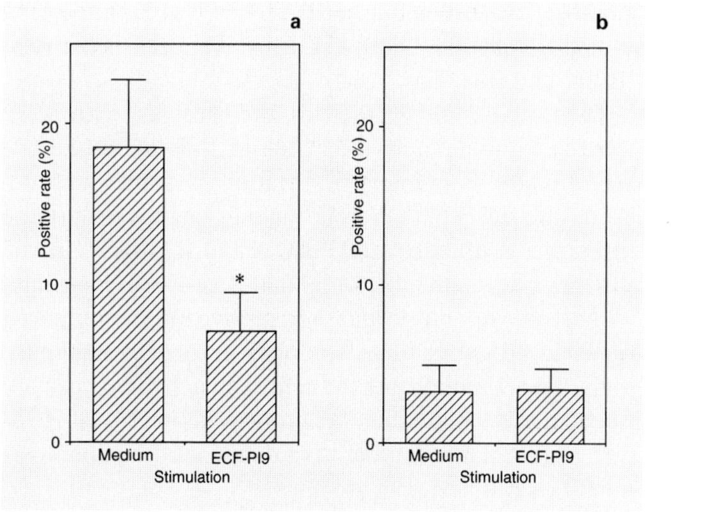

Fig. 3. Effect of ECF-PI9 on Fas expression on PB-Eos and BAL-Eos. Eosinophils from PB (**a**) and BAL (**b**) were cultured with or without ECF-PI9 for 24 h. The harvested cells were incubated with a monoclonal antibody directed against Fas, and analyzed on a FACScan. Data are means ± SD of four cases (* $p < 0.05$).

BAL-Eos also decreased from 10.6 to 3.2% (fig. 2c, d). In contrast, the percentage of viable cell of both groups increased by stimulation with ECF-PI9. The percentage of viable cells in ECF-PI9-treated PB-Eos increased from 40.1 to 60.1%, and that of the treated BAL-Eos increased from 68.0 to 80.9%. Such survival-enhancing effects of ECF-PI9 on BAL-Eos continued and started to be more apparent after 7 days' culture. Indeed, the survival rate of BAL-Eos cultured with ECF-PI9 was 65.0%, whereas that of those cultured without ECF-PI9 was only 12.2%. We also found that eotaxin had no such enhancing effect (data not shown).

Fas antigen expression on PB-Eos significantly increased from 7.2 to 17.5% after having been cultured for 1 day ($p < 0.05$), whereas that on BAL-Eos did not (from 5.2 to 3.5%). As shown in figure 3, this increase of Fas expression in PB-Eos was significantly suppressed by stimulation with ECF-PI9. In contrast, that in BAL-Eos was not suppressed by the stimulation (fig. 3).

We also attempted to isolate ECF from BAL fluid. BAL fluid exhibited evident ECF activity; its molecular weight was about 5–6 kD, and its isoelectric point was about pH 9.0. We found that this ECF isolated from BAL fluid could suppress apoptosis of both PB-Eos and BAL-Eos. The percentage of apoptotic cells in PB-Eos decreased from 33.7 to 20.5% with ECF from BAL fluid stimulation, and that of BAL-Eos also decreased from 10.6 to 4.5%, suggesting the possible involvement of ECF-PI9 in the eosinophil increase in the alveolar space in CEP.

Discussion

We described that eosinophils from PB from patients with CEP differed from those from BAL from the same patients regarding apoptosis. The survival rate of the BAL-Eos after 3 days' culture was significantly higher than that of the PB-Eos (fig. 1). This is probably the result of a decrease in the number of apoptotic cells in BAL-Eos compared to PB-Eos (fig. 2). One of the STO-2-derived ECF, ECF-PI9, suppressed the apoptosis of both PB-Eos and BAL-Eos. In addition, Fas seems to be involved in the apoptosis of PB-Eos but not BAL-Eos (fig. 3), indicating some difference in the mechanisms of apoptosis between PB-Eos and BAL-Eos.

The number of PB-Eos in the patients with CEP decreases immediately after steroid therapy, while the resolution of pulmonary infiltration is sometimes delayed. This delay of the resolution may be the result of the difference in apoptosis of PB-Eos and BAL-Eos. In the present experiments, we found that BAL-Eos are less likely to become apoptotic and they survive longer compared to PB-Eos. Most of the eosinophils in the alveolar space are in the activated state [6], and such activated cells are expected to decrease their apoptotic function [8, 9]. However, the available comparative data regarding apoptosis in PB-Eos and BAL-Eos are limited.

Eosinophil apoptosis is suspected to be related to Fas antigen [10–12]. In the present study, we found that the apoptosis of PB-Eos is correlated with the expression of Fas antigen on the cell surface (fig. 3). In contrast, the expression of Fas antigen on BAL-Eos did not change during the culture, though the apoptosis of BAL-Eos was suppressed by stimulation with ECF-PI9 (fig. 2, 3). The results of the present study indicate that the apoptosis of PB-Eos is related to the Fas antigen, whereas that of BAL-Eos is not. This is the first description showing the possibility of a difference in apoptosis between PB-Eos and BAL-Eos, though further study is needed for confirmation.

The increased production of IL-5 seems to be one of the critical pathophysiological features of eosinophilic pneumonia [4, 5]. In the light of the present results, the possibility that ECF-PI9 is also involved in the pathogenesis of CEP cannot be excluded. We have previously shown that ECF-PI9 is a potent ECF, and the chemotactic response of eosinophils to ECF-PI9 is a useful tool for examining the heterogeneity of eosinophils in CEP [1, 2]. It is clear that ECF-PI9 is not only a chemotactic factor but also an enhancing factor for eosinophil survival. We have also shown that a factor resembling ECF-PI9 can be isolated from CEP BAL fluid after isoelectric focusing; the factor with an isoelectric point of about pH 9 exhibits both eosinophil chemotactic activity and a suppressive effect on eosinophil apoptosis. It is, therefore, conceivable that ECF-PI9 is one of the factors involved in the pathogenesis of CEP. Moreover, the survival of PB-Eos from 5 patients with bronchial asthma was not enhanced by stimulation with ECF-PI9. The percentage of viable cells in ECF-PI9-treated PB-Eos changed from 13.9 to 14.2%, suggesting that PB-Eos from patients with CEP might be functionally different from PB-Eos from bronchial asthma patients.

References

1 Saita N, Hirayama S, Sugimoto M, Ando M, Hirashima M: Chemotactic heterogeneity of eosinophils in idiopathic pulmonary eosinophilia. Int Arch Allergy Immunol 1995; 108(suppl):25–27.

2 Saita N, Yamanaka T, Sugimoto M, Kohrogi H, Suga M, Ando M, Hirashima M: Heterogeneity of eosinophils in chronic eosinophilic pneumonia. Int Arch Allergy Immunol 1996; 111(suppl):29–31.

3 Carrington CB, Addlington WW, Goff AM, Madoff IM, Marks A, Schwaber JR, Gaensler EA: Chronic eosinophilic pneumonia. N Engl J Med 1969;280:787–798.

4 Kita H, Surg S, Hunt LW, Edell ES, Weiler DA, Swanson MC, Samsel RW, Abrams JS, Gleich GJ: Cytokine production at the site of disease in chronic eosinophilic pneumonia. Am J Respir Crit Care Med 1996;153:1437–1441.

5 Ino-oka N, Inoue A, Shindoh Y, Suzuki T, Konishi K: Chronic eosinophilic pneumonia associated with high concentrations of interleukin-5, -6, and granulocyte colony stimulating factor in serum and in pleural fluid (in Japanese). Nippon Kyobu Shikkan Gakkai Zasshi 1997;35:867–872.

6 Nishikawa K, Morii T, Ako H, Hamada K, Saito S, Narita N: In vivo expression of CD69 on lung eosinophils in eosinophilic pneumonia: CD69 as a possible activation marker for eosinophils. J Allergy Clin Immunol 1992;90:169–174.

7 Saita N, Yamanaka T, Kohrogi H, Matsumoto M, Suga M, Ando M, Hirashima M: Expression of apoptosis-related antigen on eosinophils in chronic eosinophilic pneumonia. Int Arch Allergy Immunol 1997;114:64–66.

8 Whyte MKB, Hardwick SJ, Meagher L, Savill J, Haslett C: Transient elevations of cytosolic free calcium retard subsequent apoptosis in neutrophils in vitro. J Clin Invest 1993;92: 446–455.

9 Woolley KL, Gibson PG, Carty K, Wilson AJ, Twaddell SH, Woolley MJ: Eosinophil apoptosis and the resolution of airway inflammation in asthma. Am J Respir Crit Care Med 1996; 154:237–243.

10 Matsumoto K, Schleimer RP, Saito H, Iikura Y, Bochner Y: Induction of apoptosis in human eosinophils by anti-Fas antibody treatment in vitro. Blood 1995;96:1447–1453.

11 Luttmann W, Opfer A, Dauer E, Forester M, Matthys H, Eibel H, Schulze-Osthoff K, Kroegel C, Virchow JC: Differential regulation of CD95 (Fas/APO-1) expression in human blood eosinophils. Eur J Immunol 1998;28:2057–2065.

12 Druilhe A, Cai Z, Haile S, Chouaib S, Pretolani M: Fas-mediated apoptosis in cultured human eosinophils. Blood 1996;87:2822–2830.

13 Levi-Schaffer F, Temkin V, Malamud V, Feld S, Zilberman Y: Mast cells enhance eosinophil survival in vitro: Role of TNF-alpha and granulocyte-macrophage colony-stimulating factor. J Immunol 1998;160:5554–5562.

International Archives of
Allergy and
Immunology

Int Arch Allergy Immunol 1999;120(suppl 1):95–99

Circadian Variation in Nasal Reactivity in Children with Allergic Rhinitis: Correlation with the Activity of Eosinophils and Basophilic Cells

Masahiko Aoyagi[a] Hiroko Watanabe[a] Kunio Sekine[a] Toshiyuki Nishimuta[a]
Akiyoshi Konno[b] Naoki Shimojo[c] Yoichi Kohno[c]

[a]Department of Pediatrics and Clinical Research, National Shimoshizu Hospital, Yotsukaido, Chiba, and
Departments of [b]Otorhinolaryngology and [c]Pediatrics, School of Medicine, Chiba University, Chiba, Japan

Key Words
Nasal reactivity · Circadian variation · Eosinophil cationic protein · Histamine · Tryptase

Abstract
Background: In allergic rhinitis, the major symptoms of runny nose, sneezing, and stuffy nose tend to become worse upon waking up in the morning, and yet the mechanisms underlying this phenomenon are poorly understood. We investigated whether the worsening of allergic rhinitis in the morning is associated with changes in the activity of inflammatory cells. ***Methods:*** Nasal reactivity to methacholine was assessed twice in 8 children with allergic rhinitis and 8 healthy control subjects at 6.00 a.m. and 3.00 p.m. The amounts of eosinophil cationic protein (ECP), histamine and tryptase in induced nasal secretions and peripheral blood were also measured. ***Results:*** Nasal reactivity to methacholine was higher at 6.00 a.m. not only in patients but also in healthy controls. Serum ECP and plasma histamine levels showed no circadian patterns. On the other hand, significantly higher levels of inflammatory activation products were found in nasal secretions at 6.00 a.m., thus showing a direct association with nasal reactivity. ***Conclusion:*** These results suggest that the circadian variation in nasal reactivity is associated with changes in the activity of eosinophils and basophilic cells in the nasal mucosa.

Introduction

The symptoms of allergic disorders of the respiratory tract exhibit a circadian rhythm. Nocturnal and morning dyspnea in asthma [1–3] and worsening of allergic rhinitis in the morning are very common. Many studies have focussed on the mechanisms of nocturnal asthma [4–8], but little is known about allergic rhinitis.

Nasal reactivity in allergic rhinitis is closely related to allergic inflammation, particularly to infiltration by activated eosinophils and basophilic cells in the nasal mucosa [9, 10]. Repeated antigenic challenges in subjects with allergic rhinitis enhance the infiltration of these inflammatory cells in the nasal mucosa and enhance nasal reactivity [11]. We hypothesized that the numbers of activated inflammatory cells in the nasal mucosa would increase in the morning and that these changes would cause worsening in the morning. Therefore, we investigated changes in nasal reactivity and inflammatory me-

KARGER
Fax +41 61 306 12 34
E-Mail karger@karger.ch
www.karger.com

1018–2438/99/1205–0095$17.50/0

Accessible online at:
http://BioMedNet.com/karger

Masahiko Aoyagi, MD
Department of Pediatrics and Clinical Research
National Shimoshizu Hospital, 934-5 Shikawatashi
Yotsukaido, Chiba 284-0003 (Japan)
Tel. +81 43 422 2511, Fax +81 43 421 3007, E-Mail cfy27505@simosizu.hosp.go.jp

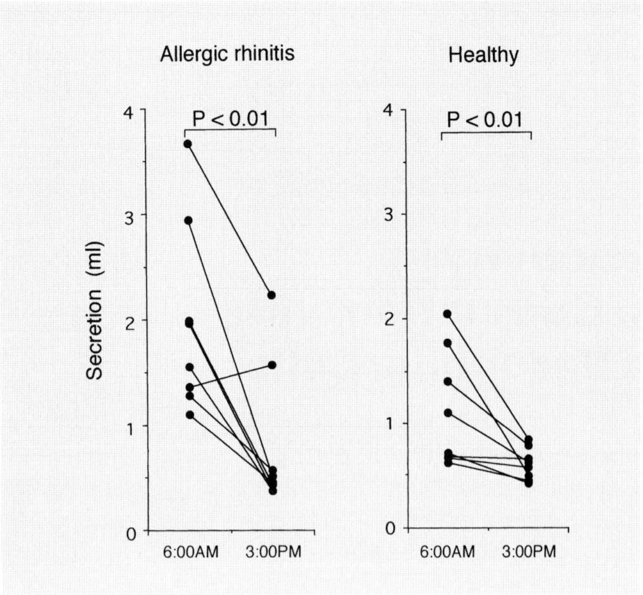

Fig. 1. Changes in nasal reactivity. Nasal reactivity to methacholine was increased at 6.00 a.m. not only in patients but also in healthy controls.

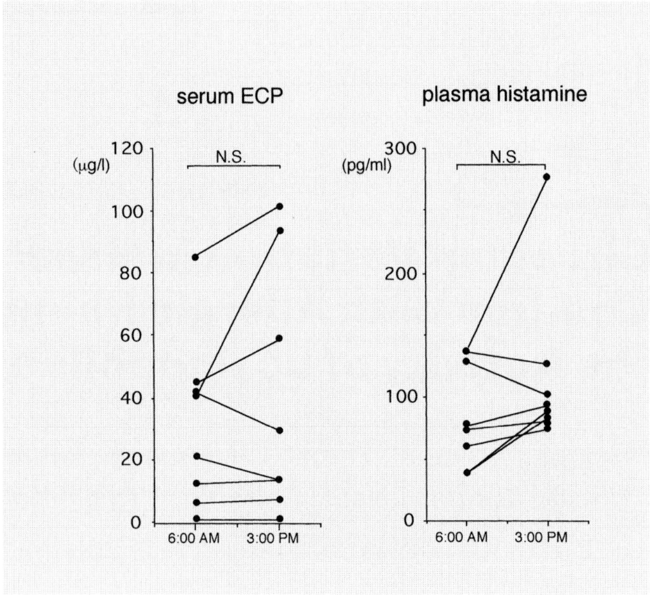

Fig. 2. Changes in serum ECP and plasma histamine levels. Serum ECP and plasma histamine levels showed no circadian patterns in agreement with nasal reactivity.

diators [eosinophil cationic protein (ECP), histamine and tryptase] in induced nasal secretions and peripheral blood, and discuss their relationship with nasal reactivity.

Materials and Methods

Patients

Eight allergic donors (6 males, 2 females) represented the patients with allergic rhinitis aged 9–14 years (mean age 11.3 ± 2.2 years). As controls, 8 age-matched normal donors without a history of allergic disease were selected. All patients had refrained from using nasal and oral corticosteroids, antiallergic drugs and antihistamines for at least 2 weeks before nasal challenge. The symptom scores during 2 weeks before challenge were recorded; the degree of nasal congestion, rhinorrhea and sneezing was graded by each patient on a scale of 0–3, where none = 0, mild = 1, moderate = 2 and severe = 3. Furthermore, a composite symptom score was calculated as the sum of the scores for nasal congestion, rhinorrhea and sneezing.

Methacholine Challenge and Collection of Nasal Secretion

Nasal challenge was performed at 6.00 a.m. and 3.00 p.m. by spraying 12 mg methacholine at a concentration of 130 mg/ml into each nasal cavity and then collecting for 10 min the resulting secretion which dripped into a polyethylene sack while the subject bent his head forward. The volume of secretion was calculated from the weight and the specific gravity of the secretion. Nasal secretions from each patient were diluted 4-fold with phosphate-buffered saline containing 0.3% EDTA. The diluted sample was vortexed, centrifuged at 4,400 *g* for 10 min at 0 °C, and the supernatant was collected and stored at –20 °C until used.

Determination of ECP, Histamine and Tryptase

ECP and tryptase concentrations in nasal secretions and serum were measured by radioimmunoassays (RIA) (Pharmacia Diagnostics, Uppsala, Sweden) as described previously [12]. The detection level in the assay was 2 ng/ml. The histamine level in secretions and plasma was measured by RIA (Immunotech, Westbrook, Me., USA) according to the manufacturer's protocol. The detection level in the assay was 50 pg/ml. The amounts of inflammatory mediators in the induced secretions were shown by the net amount (the mediator concentration × volume of nasal secretion).

Statistics

The Wilcoxon signed rank test was used to compare nasal reactivity, ECP, histamine and tryptase at 6.00 a.m. and 3.00 p.m. Correlations between inflammatory mediators and nasal reactivity were calculated with the Pearson correlation.

Results

Nasal Reactivity

We evaluated mucosal reactivity by the volume of methacholine-induced nasal secretion. Figure 1 demonstrates the nasal reactivity to methacholine at 6.00 a.m. and 3.00 p.m. In patients with allergic rhinitis, nasal reactivity was significantly increased at 6.00 a.m., and these

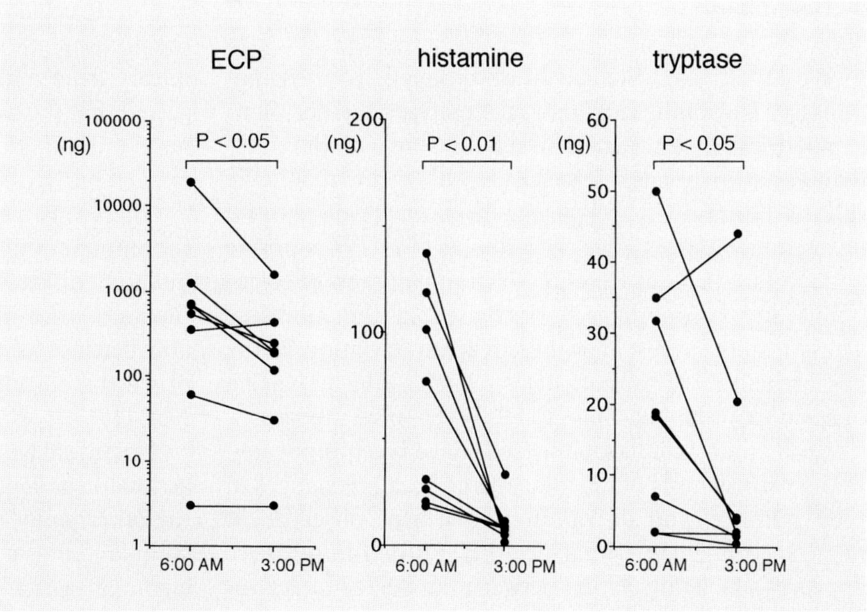

Fig. 3. Changes in the amounts of ECP, histamine and tryptase in nasal secretions. The levels of these inflammatory mediators were significantly higher in nasal secretions at 6.00 a.m.

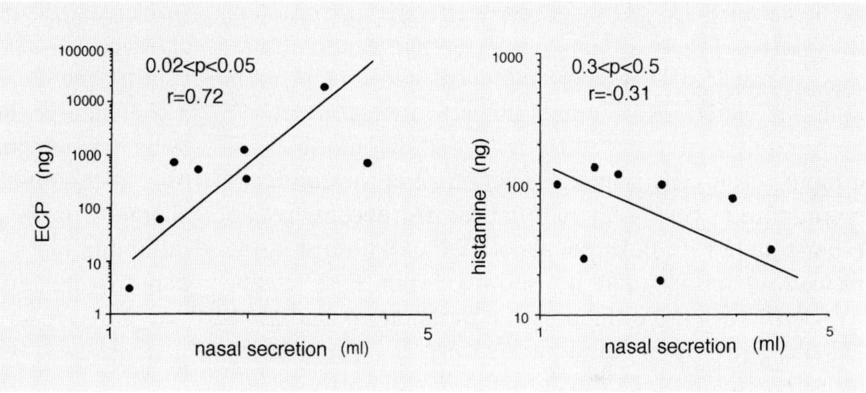

Fig. 4. Correlation between inflammatory mediators in nasal secretions and nasal reactivity. The amount of ECP in the nasal secretions correlated with nasal reactivity, but the amount of histamine did not.

results correlated with their subjective symptoms. A statistical correlation was found between nasal reactivities and composite symptom scores during 2 weeks before challenge ($r = 0.52$; $0.02 < p < 0.05$). The changes in nasal reactivity were similar in patients and healthy controls with no symptom of rhinitis.

Circadian Variation of Inflammatory Mediators in Subjects with Allergic Rhinitis

Serum ECP and plasma histamine levels showed no circadian patterns in agreement with nasal reactivity (fig. 2). Furthermore, no significant variations in peripheral eosinophil counts between 6.00 a.m. and 3.00 p.m. were found (data not shown).

The amounts of inflammatory mediators in the induced secretions are shown in figure 3. The amounts of ECP in the secretions were significantly increased in the morning, and the amounts of histamine and tryptase showed the same pattern as ECP.

Correlations between Mediators and Nasal Symptoms

A weak correlation occurred between the amounts of histamine and the degrees of rhinorrhea or sneezing, but no significant correlation was observed between the amounts of ECP or tryptase and nasal symptoms (data not shown).

Correlations with Nasal Reactivity

The amounts of ECP in nasal secretions at 6.00 a.m. correlated significantly with nasal reactivity, but the amounts of histamine did not (fig. 4, analyses were performed on the logarithmic transformation).

Discussion

We investigated the activation products from eosinophils and basophilic cells in nasal secretions and peripheral blood, and determined their relationship with the circadian variation of nasal reactivity in children with allergic rhinitis. Serum ECP and plasma histamine levels showed no circadian patterns, but the amounts of ECP, histamine and tryptase in nasal secretions, activity markers of eosinophils and basophilic cells increased in the morning. These results suggest that the circadian variation in the nasal reactivity of the patients is related to the activation of eosinophils and basophilic cells in the nasal mucosa.

Eosinophils and basophilic cells have been implicated in the pathogenesis of mucosal allergy because changes in their numbers and distribution have been observed in relation to allergen stimulation [9]. Furthermore, there appears to be a correlation between the degree of activation of these inflammatory cells and nasal symptoms or nasal reactivity [13]. Our data show circadian variation in the activity of these inflammatory cells in the nasal mucosa. Ohtsuka et al. [14] reported that basophilic cell counts in nasal secretions of atopic subjects increased in the morning. We did not directly count the numbers of inflammatory cells in nasal secretions, but the counts of eosinophils or basophilic cells in the brush specimens did not correlate with the amounts of ECP or with histamine in nasal secretions (data not shown). From these results, we speculate that the amounts of inflammatory mediators depend not only on the total number of inflammatory cells but also on the activity of inflammatory cells.

What regulates the circadian variation in the activity of inflammatory cells? Several investigators have suggested that the autonomic central nervous system plays a role in the development of nocturnal airway obstruction [4, 6, 7]. Certainly, allergen exposure at night may have an effect on the activation of mucosal inflammatory cells in the morning. But we consider too that an autonomic circadian rhythm is more important rather than this, because circadian variation in nasal reactivity is observed not only in patients but also in healthy controls. Thus, we measured adrenaline and noradrenaline concentrations in the peripheral blood of healthy controls. There was a fall in the levels of circulating adrenaline and noradrenaline in the morning (data not shown). Our observations are consistent with the findings of Barnes et al. [4], who observed a morning decrease of plasma adrenaline concentration in patients with asthma. The autonomic circadian rhythm influences the axon reflex, and circulating adrenaline and noradrenaline could act on eosinophils and mast cells by stimulating β-adrenoceptors to inhibit the accumulation of eosinophils [15, 16] and histamine release from mast cells and basophils [17, 18]. It is suggested that the circadian variation in nasal reactivity and nasal inflammatory cells may be caused by the autonomic circadian rhythm.

There was a correlation between nasal reactivity and the amount of ECP in the nasal secretions in the morning, but no significant correlation between nasal reactivity and the amount of histamine was observed. This is presumably because we evaluated nasal reactivity by the volume of nasal secretion, which is more directly influenced by ECP [19].

Nocturnal worsening of asthma is common, but not all asthmatic patients show nocturnal airway obstruction. On the other hand, most patients with allergic rhinitis have complained of a worsening in the morning. In addition, circadian variation in nasal reactivity is observed in patients and healthy controls. Although we did not measure mediators in the secretions of healthy controls, several investigators reported that in patients with allergic rhinitis, the ECP and tryptase level in nasal secretion was higher than in healthy controls [20–22]. These observations may support our hypothesis that a circadian variation in the nasal reactivity is common in patients with allergic rhinitis and healthy subjects; however, allergic inflammation in patients enhances the autonomic circadian rhythm and nasal symptoms.

References

1 Reinberg A, Gervais P, Levi F, Smolensky M, Del Cerro L, Ugolini C: Circadian and circannual rhythms of allergic rhinitis: An epidemiologic study involving chronobiologic methods. J Allergy Clin Immunol 1988;81:51–62.

2 Smolensky MH, Reinberg A, Labrecque G: Twenty-four hour pattern in symptom intensity of viral and allergic rhinitis: Treatment implications. J Allergy Clin Immunol 1995;95: 1084–1096.

3 Turner-Warwick M: Epidemiology of nocturnal asthma. Am J Med 1988;85:1B:6–8.

4 Barnes P, Fitzgerald G, Brown M, Dollery C: Nocturnal asthma and changes in circulating epinephrine, histamine, and cortisol. N Engl J Med 1980;303:263–267.

5 Martin RJ, Cicutto LC, Smith HR, Ballard RD, Szefler SJ: Airway inflammation in nocturnal asthma. Am Rev Respir Dis 1991;143: 351–357.

6 van Aalderen, Postma DS, Koëter GH, Knol K: Nocturnal airflow obstruction, histamine, and the autonomic central nervous system in children with allergic asthma. Thorax 1991;46: 366–371.

7 Bates ME, Clayton M; Calhoun W, Jarjour N, Schrader L, Geiger K, Schultz T, Sedgwick J, Swenson C, Busse W: Relationship of plasma epinephrine and circulating eosinophils to nocturnal asthma. Am J Respir Crit Care Med 1994;149:667–672.

8 Oosterhoff Y, Hoogsteden HC, Rutgers B, Kauffman HF, Postma DS: Lymphocyte and macrophage activation in bronchoalveolar lavage fluid in nocturnal asthma. Am J Respir Crit Care Med 1995;151:75–81.

9 Juliusson S, Pipkorn U, Karlsson G, Enerbäck L: Mast cells and eosinophils in the allergic mucosal response to allergen challenge: Changes in distribution and signs of activation in relation to symptoms. J Allergy Clin Immunol 1992;90:898–909.

10 Konno A, Yamakoshi T, Terada N, Fujita Y: Mode of action of a topical steroid on immediate phase reaction after antigen challenge and nonspecific nasal hyperreactivity in nasal allergy. Int Arch Allergy Immunol 1994;103:79–87.

11 Pipkorn U, Karlsson G, Enerbäck L: Nasal mucosal response to repeated challenges with pollen allergen. Am Rev Respir Dis 1989;140: 729–736.

12 Peterson CGB, Enander I, Nystrand J, Anderson AS, Nilsson L, Venge P: Radioimmunoassay of human eosinophil cationic protein (ECP) by an improved method: Establishment of normal levels in serum and turnover in vivo. Clin Exp Allergy 1991;21:561–567.

13 Ohtsuka H, Okuda M: Basophilic cells in allergic nasal secretions. Part III. Jibika-Rinshoh 1978;71:1085–1096.

14 Pipkorn U, Karlsson G, Enerbäck L: The cellular response of the human allergic mucosa to natural allergen exposure. J Allergy Clin Immunol 1988;86:1046–1054.

15 Hadjokas NE, Crowley JJ, Bayer CR, Nielson CP: β-Adrenergic regulation of the eosinophil respiratory burst as detected by lucigenin-dependent luminescence. J Allergy Clin Immunol 1995;95:735–741.

16 Teixeira MM, Hellewell PG: Evidence that the eosinophil is a cellular target for the inhibitory action of salmeterol on eosinophil recruitment in vivo. Eur J Pharmacol 1997;323:255–260.

17 Church MK, Hiroi J: Inhibition of IgE-dependent histamine release from human dispersed lung mast cells by anti-allergic drugs and salbutamol. Br J Pharmacol 1987;90:421–429.

18 Barnes PJ: Endoegnous catecholamines and asthma. J Allergy Clin Immunol 1986;77:791–795.

19 Lundgen JD, Davey RT Jr, Lundgren B, Mullol J, Marom Z, Longun C, Baraniuk J, Kaliner MA, Shelhamer JH: Eosinophil cationic protein stimulates and major basic protein inhibits airway mucus secretion. J Allergy Clin Immunol 1991;87:689–698.

20 Beppu T, Ohta N, Gon S, Sakata K, Inamura K, Fukase S, Kimura Y, Koike Y: Eosinophil and eosinophil cationic protein in allergic rhinitis. Acta Otolaryngol Suppl (Stockh) 1994;511: 221–223.

21 Rasp G, Bujia J: Diagnosis of allergic rhinitis by determining of tryptase and eosinophil cationic protein in nasal secretions. Acta Otorrinolaringol Esp 1994;45:437–440.

22 Klimek L, Rasp G: Cell activation markers in rhinitis and rhinosinusitis. 1. Eosinophilic cationic protein. Laryngorhinootologie 1996;75: 665–670.

International Archives of Allergy and Immunology

Int Arch Allergy Immunol 1999;120(suppl 1):100–103

Overexpression of CD11b on Eosinophils in Atopic Dermatitis: Downregulation by Cyclosporin A and Upregulation by Interleukin 5

Hidekazu Yamada[a] Shinji Kurashimo[b] Junichi Chihara[c]
Masaharu Matsukura[a] Tatsuo Yudate[a] Tadashi Tezuka[a]

[a]Department of Dermatology and [b]Life Science Research Institute, School of Medicine, Kinki University, Osaka, and [c]Department of Experimental Medicine School of Medicine, Akita University, Akita, Japan

Key Words
Eosinophils · CD11b · Flow cytometry · Interleukin 5 · Cyclosporin A

Abstract
We examined the level of expression of CD11b on eosinophils in pripheral blood samples from patients with atopic dermatitis (AD) and non-AD volunteers. Eosinophils were defined using a new method employing CD14/CD45 and a backgate technique. Overexpression of CD11b was noted in eosinophils of AD patients. Treatment of AD with cyclosporin A resulted in clinical improvement as well as reduction in the expression of CD11b. Stimulation of eosinophils from patients with inactive AD by interleukin 5 upregulated the expression of CD11b on these cells. Our results suggest that the expression of CD11b surface molecule on eosinophils may play an important role in the activity of AD.

Introduction

Eosinophils are known to function as effector cells and play an important role in the pathogenesis of allergic inflammatory reactions. Therefore, examination of the surface antigens on eosinophils is essential for our understanding of the pathogenesis of allergic disorders. CD11b is a member of the β_2 integrin family and is expressed on monocytes.

In studies on eosinophils, it is necessary to detect the nature of surface antigens by using cytometry. We used a new cytometric method to separate eosinophils and determined the expression of CD11b on these cells in patients with atopic dermatitis (AD).

Materials and Methods

Patients

The subjects in this study included 7 patients with AD and 3 control patients without AD. All AD patients had eosinophilia as determined by differential cell count in peripheral blood samples. The diagnosis and severity of AD were assessed according to the criteria of Haniffin and Rajka [1] and Rajka and Langeland [2]. In 2 patients, cyclosporin A (5 mg/kg) was used for 4 weeks for the control of AD.

Monoclonal Antibodies

A panel of monoclonal antibodies (mAbs) was selected to evaluate surface antigens on lymphocytes and eosinophils. These mAbs consisted of anti-CD14 (FITC-labeled mouse IgG1, Becton Dickinson, USA), CD45 (PE-labeled mouse IgG1, Becton Dickinson), CD11b (FITC-labeled mouse IgG1, Becton Dickinson), and CD16 (FITC-labeled mouse IgG1, Becton Dickinson). FITC-labeled mouse IgG1 and PE-labeled mouse IgG1 were used as isotype controls.

KARGER

Fax + 41 61 306 12 34
E-Mail karger@karger.ch
www.karger.com

1018–2438/99/1205–0100$17.50/0

Accessible online at:
http://BioMedNet.com/karger

Dr. Hidekazu Yamada
Department of Dermatology, School of Medicine, Kinki University
377 Ohonohigashi, Osaka-sayama, Osaka 589 (Japan)
Tel. +81 723 66 0221, ext. 3228, Fax +81 723 68 2120
E-Mail yamadahi@med.kindai.ac.jp

Fixation and Cell Staining

Cells were stained using the protocol recommended by the manufacturer. Briefly, 100 µl of whole blood was placed in a polystyrene tube (Falcon No. 2008) and cells were stained directly with fluorescence-labeled mAb at room temperature for 15 min. Red blood cells were hemolyzed by FACS Lysing Solution (Becton Dickinson) and washed with Hankgs' buffer saline solution.

Flow-Cytometric Analysis and Sorting

To analyze eosinophils, total granulocytes were gated based on a unique foreward scatter and side scatter characteristics compared with those of neutrophils. Double staining with FITC-CD14/PE-CD45 mAbs showed eosinophilic granules in the center of the field. We gated with this spot and then fluorescence gated (back-gated) to SSC/FSC. These cells represented CD16-negative clusters. To confirm the purity of eosinophil clusters identified using our method, the cell populations were sorted using venous blood samples drawn from AD patients. The sample was processed as previously described except that 500 µl of whole blood were stained with 20 µl of each of the appropriate mAb and resuspended in a final volume of 1 ml PBS with 1% paraformaldehyde in order to increase the number of cells available for sorting. Sorting was carried out on a Becton Dickinson FACS Caliber. Eosinophils were sorted by using the CD14/45 and then gated with SSC and FSC fluorescence plots and the cells collected in PBS. They were then spun down and resuspended in 100 µl RPMI with 10% fetal calf serum. A cytospin preparation was prepared from the cell population, fixed in methanol, and stained with the modified Wright-Giemsa stain for examination under light microscopy. The percentage of eosinophils expressing a specific marker was determined relative to the expression level on the isotype-negative control.

Culture Conditions

Peripheral blood samples wer collected and anticoagulated with EDTA. Eosinophils were isolated by negative selection with anti-CD16-magnetic beads using the method described by Chihara et al. [3] with some modification. Eosinophils were incubated for 24 h at 37 °C with recombinant interleukin (rIL)-5 (Genzyme, USA). Fluorescence was measured on a FACS caliber.

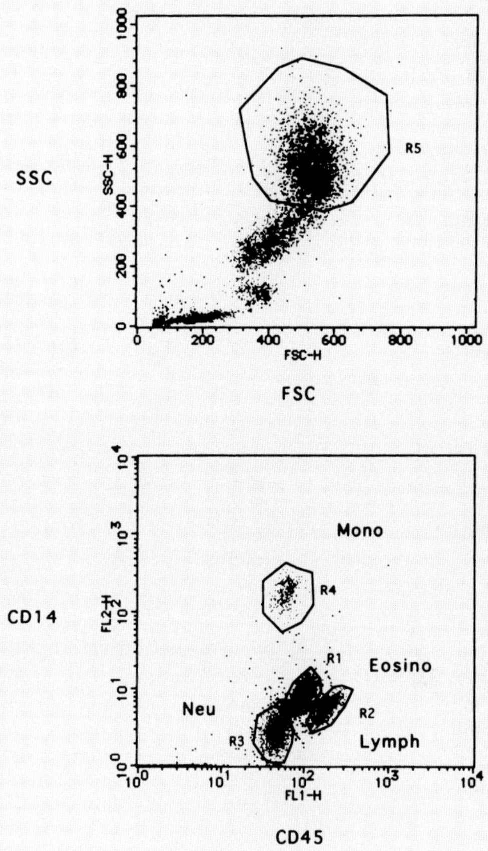

Fig. 1. Flow-cytometric characteristics of eosinophils with CD14/CD45. SSC/FSC were backgated from CD14/CD45.

Results

Identification of Eosinophils with CD14/CD45

Eosinophils were gated based on CD14/CD45 staining and forward scatter by side scatter characteristics (fig. 1). To define eosinophils, cells were sorted and eosinophils were detected based on morphological features. This analysis showed that 99.9% of the cells were eosinophils, indicating that the use of CD14/CD15 is useful for the separation of eosinophils in FACS analysis.

CD11b Overexpression on Eosinophils in AD

We used the new method for separation of eosinophils, and the surface molecules on eosinophils were stained by anti-CD11b. The percentages of positive cells are shown in table 1. The percentage of CD11b-positive cells was

Table 1. Percentage of eosinophils in peripheral blood samples and expression of CD11b on these cells in patients with atopic dermatitis and control subjects

Severity of AD	Eosinophils, %	Positive CD11b, %
Severe	17	86.9
Severe	23	88.1
Severe	31	99.7
Moderate	15	93.9
Moderate	12	98.9
Moderate	8	75.3
Moderate	9	97.2
Mean ± SD		91.4 ± 8.1
Non-AD	3	51.9
Non-AD	4	63.9
Non-AD	2	49.0
Mean ± SD		54.9 ± 6.4

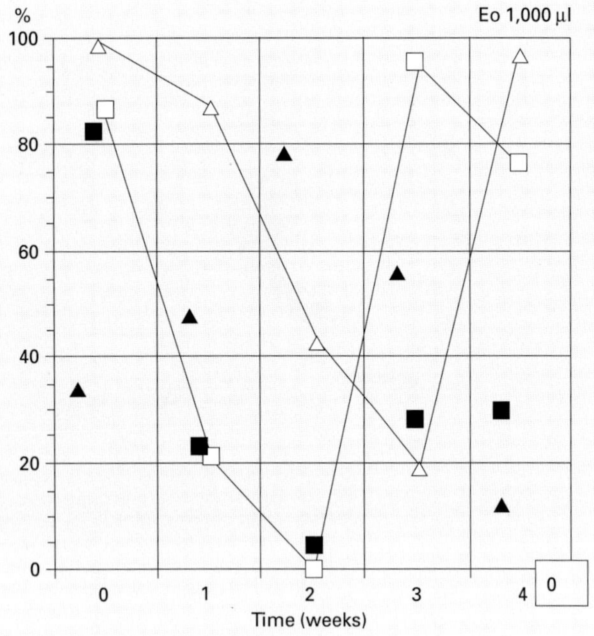

Fig. 2. Serial changes in CD11b expression on eosinophils in 2 patients with AD treated with cyclosporin A: numbers of eosinophils (counts/µl) in patient OT (■) and patient KH (▲) and CD11b-positive eosinophils (1,000/µl) in patient OT (□) and patient KH (△).

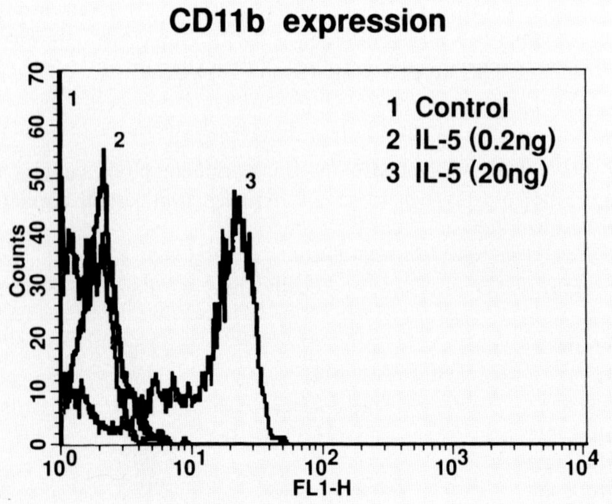

Fig. 3. CD11b upregulation on eosinophils from patients with non-active AD with IL-5. Eosinophils were cultured with IL-5 for 12 h.

high in all 7 patients with AD and was significantly different compared to that in healthy control.

Cyclosporin A Downregulates CD11b (fig. 2).

Two patients with AD were treated with cyclosporin A to reduce eosinophilia and skin eruptions. Figure 2 shows the serial changes in CD11b during this treatment. Administration of oral cyclosporin A downregulated CD11b, in association with an amelioration of skin eruptions within 2 weeks. However, the percentage of CD11b-positive eosinophils increased 3 weeks later. This change was not associated with changes in the skin condition.

IL-5 Upregulates CD11b on Eosinophils in vitro

Flow cytometry experiments were performed to determine whether cytokines are involved in the upregulation of CD11b. Preincubation of eosinophils with rIL-5 resulted in the upregulation of CD11b (fig. 3). The results also showed that this effect was dose-dependent.

Discussion

Identification of eosinophils in whole blood samples by flow cytometry can be problematic because eosinophils overlap significantly with neutrophil clusters on forward scatter versus side scatter plots of whole blood samples. In this study, we used leukogate for lymphocytes and detected eosinophil clusters of mild intensities in fluorescence of the CD14/CD45. Using the backgate technique, eosinophils were detected in the FSC/SSC screen. Gopinath and Nutman [4] have recently described a new method to detect eosinophil clusters by using high side scatter and CD16-negative selection. In the same year, Enokihara et al. [5] used the characteristics of eosinophils to identify these cells by their autofluorescence-positive granulocytes and then determined them by flow cytometry. With our method, we also attempted to measure the sensitivity of eosinophil sorting. The results showed that 99.9% of the cells were eosinophils. These results indicate that CD14/CD45 leukogate staining and the backgate method are also useful for distinguishing eosinophils form lysed blood cells.

Using this method, we separated the eosinophils in the sample and measured the surface markers on their surface in patients with AD. In the present study, cytometry was performed after staining cells in whole blood samples to avoid the risk of purification-based activation. Comparison of eosinophils from patients with AD with those from normal individuals showed a significantly higher expression of CD11b expression on these cells in AD. Such overexpression of CD11b is likely to explain, at least in part, the differences in eosinophil function in AD. To further confirm the involvement of CD11b on eosinophils in AD, we examined the effects of cyclosporin A on this surface marker of eosinophils in 2 representative patients with AD. A 2-week treatment using this agent resulted in an improvement of the skin condition, which was associated with a downregulation of CD11b on eosinophils [6–8]. From the data of eosinophil numbers after 3 weeks' treatment, it is possible that eosinophila expressing CD11b is resistant to cyclosporin. Hakansson et al. [9] and others [10, 11] showed that the CD11b expression of eosinophils from asthma is high. The mechanism of infiltration and degranulation for eosinophils in blood may be common in atopic diseases like asthma and AD. These results also indicate that the level of expression of CD11b is clinically useful as a marker for eosinophil activity at least in patients with AD. Several studies [12, 13] have shown that the level of CD11b expression on eosinophils is influenced by a variety of cytokines such as IL-5 and GM-CSF.

To confirm the involvement of such cytokines in AD, we also examined the effect of rIL-5 on eosinophils from patients with an inactive stage of AD on the expression of CD11b. Our data showed that rIL-5 increased dose-dependently the level of CD11b expression on eosinophils. These results clearly showed that CD11b expression on eosinophils is dependent on IL-5. Our results also suggested that in patients with active AD, CD11b expression on eosinophils may be upregulated by IL-5 in the peripheral blood.

In conclusion, we described a novel method for sorting eosinophils in peripheral blood samples. Using this method, we showed a high expression of CD11b on eosinophils of patients with active dermatitis, which diminished following treatment with cyclosporin A. Furthermore, we also showed that such an overexpression of CD11b is upregulated, at least in part, by IL-5.

References

1 Haniffin MJ, Rajka G: Diagnostic features of atopic dermatitis. Acta Derm Venereol 1980; 92:44–47.
2 Rajka G, Langeland T: Grading of the severity of atopic dermatitis. Acta Derm Venereol 1989;144:13–14.
3 Chihara J, Kurachi D, Yamamoto T, Yamada H, Wada T, Yasukawa A, Nakajima S: A comparative study of eosinophil isolation by different procedures of CD16-negative depletion. Allergy 1995;50:11–14.
4 Gopinath R, Nutman TB: Identification of eosinophils in lysed whole blood using side scatter and CD16 negativity. Cytometry 1997;30: 313–316.
5 Enokihara H, Koike T, Nakamura Y, Saito K, Furusawa S: Identification of surface molecules on eosinophils and lymphocytes in blood from patients with eosinophilia. Int Arch Allergy Immunol 1997;114(suppl 1):72–74.
6 Ebisawa M, Bochner BS, Georas SN, Schleimer RP: Eosinophil transendothelial migration induced by cytokines. I. Role of endothelial and eosinophil adhesion molecules in IL-1 beta-induced transendothelial migration. J Immunol 1992;149:4021–4028.
7 Spoelstra FM, Hovenga H, Noordhoek JA, Postma DS, Kauffman HF: Change sin CD11b and L-selectin expression on eosinophils are mediated by human lung fibroblasts in vitro. Am J Respir Crit Care Med 1998;158:769–777.
8 Walsh GM, Hartnell A, Wardlaw AJ, Kurihara K, Sanderson CJ, Kay AB: IL-5 enhances the in vitro adhesion of human eosinophils, but not neutrophils, in a leucocyte integrin (CD11/18)-dependent manner. Immunology 1990;71: 258–265.
9 Hakansson L, Bjornsson E, Janson C, Schmekel B: Increased adhesion to vascular cell adhesion molecule-1 and intercellular adhesion molecule-1 of eosinophils from patients with asthma. J Allergy Clin Immunol 1995;96:941–950.
10 Hartnell A, Moqbel R, Walsh GM, Bradley B, Kay AB: Fc gamma and CD11/CD18 receptor expression on normal density and low density human eosinophils. Immunolgy 1990;69:264–270.
11 Fernvik E, Gronneberg R, Lundahl J, Hed J, Andersson O, Johansson SG, Hallden G: The degree of natural allergen exposure modifies eosinophil activity markers in the circulation of patients with mild asthma. Allergy 1996;51: 697–705.
12 Horie S, Kita H: CD11b/CD18 (Mac-1) is required for degranulation of human eosinophils induced by human recombinant granulocyte-macrophage colony-stimulating factor and platelet-activating factor. J Immunol 1994;152: 5457–5467.
13 in 't Venn JC, Grootendorst DC, Bel EH, Smits HH, Van Der Keur M, Sterk PJ, Hiemstra PS: CD11b and L-selectin expression on eosinophils and neutrophils in blood and induced sputum of patients with asthma compared with normal subjects. Clin Exp Allergy 1998;28: 606–615.

Author Index Vol. 120, Suppl. 1, 1999

International Archives of Allergy and Immunology

KARGER

Fax + 41 61 306 12 34
E-Mail karger@karger.ch
www.karger.com

Accessible online at:
http://BioMedNet.com/karger

International Archives of
Allergy and Immunology

Subject Index Vol. 120, Suppl. 1, 1999

KARGER
Fax +41 61 306 12 34
E-Mail karger@karger.ch
www.karger.com

Accessible online at:
http://BioMedNet.com/karger